GENETICS - RESEARCH AND ISSUES

FRAGILE X SYNDROME

FROM DIAGNOSIS TO TREATMENT

GENETICS - RESEARCH AND ISSUES

Additional books and e-books in this series can be found
on Nova's website under the Series tab.

Genetics - Research and Issues

Fragile X Syndrome

From Diagnosis to Treatment

Fabrizio Stasolla
Editor

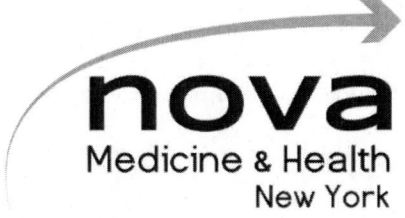

Copyright © 2022 by Nova Science Publishers, Inc.
DOI: https://doi.org/10.52305/KEUN5004

All rights reserved. No part of this book may be reproduced, stored in a retrieval system or transmitted in any form or by any means: electronic, electrostatic, magnetic, tape, mechanical photocopying, recording or otherwise without the written permission of the Publisher.

We have partnered with Copyright Clearance Center to make it easy for you to obtain permissions to reuse content from this publication. Simply navigate to this publication's page on Nova's website and locate the "Get Permission" button below the title description. This button is linked directly to the title's permission page on copyright.com. Alternatively, you can visit copyright.com and search by title, ISBN, or ISSN.

For further questions about using the service on copyright.com, please contact:
Copyright Clearance Center
Phone: +1-(978) 750-8400   Fax: +1-(978) 750-4470   E-mail: info@copyright.com.

NOTICE TO THE READER

The Publisher has taken reasonable care in the preparation of this book, but makes no expressed or implied warranty of any kind and assumes no responsibility for any errors or omissions. No liability is assumed for incidental or consequential damages in connection with or arising out of information contained in this book. The Publisher shall not be liable for any special, consequential, or exemplary damages resulting, in whole or in part, from the readers' use of, or reliance upon, this material. Any parts of this book based on government reports are so indicated and copyright is claimed for those parts to the extent applicable to compilations of such works.

Independent verification should be sought for any data, advice or recommendations contained in this book. In addition, no responsibility is assumed by the Publisher for any injury and/or damage to persons or property arising from any methods, products, instructions, ideas or otherwise contained in this publication.

This publication is designed to provide accurate and authoritative information with regard to the subject matter covered herein. It is sold with the clear understanding that the Publisher is not engaged in rendering legal or any other professional services. If legal or any other expert assistance is required, the services of a competent person should be sought. FROM A DECLARATION OF PARTICIPANTS JOINTLY ADOPTED BY A COMMITTEE OF THE AMERICAN BAR ASSOCIATION AND A COMMITTEE OF PUBLISHERS.

Additional color graphics may be available in the e-book version of this book.

Library of Congress Cataloging-in-Publication Data

ISBN: 978-1-68507-572-9

Published by Nova Science Publishers, Inc. † New York

To my mother

Contents

Preface ix

Chapter 1 **Fragile X Syndrome: Pathological Mechanisms and Molecular Bases**............................1
Mónica Alejandra Rosales-Reynoso,
Anilú Margarita Saucedo-Sariñana,
Mariana Pérez-Coria and Patricio Barros-Núñez

Chapter 2 **Fragile X Syndrome: Common Neuropsychiatric Associations**...................43
Silvina Tonarelli and Zarin Akhter

Chapter 3 **Pharmacotherapy of Fragile X Syndrome**................61
Maria Jimena Salcedo-Arellano,
Ramkumar Aishworiya, Randi Hagerman
and Dragana Protic

Chapter 4 **General Features and Conceptual Issues on Fragile X Syndrome**...................................93
Donatella Ciarmoli and Fabrizio Stasolla

Chapter 5 **Microswitch-Cluster Technology to Promote Constructive Engagement and Reduce Mouthing in Two Children with Fragile X Syndrome and Developmental Disabilities**.............111
Donatella Ciarmoli and Fabrizio Stasolla

Chapter 6	**Microswitch and VOCA to Independently Access Positive Stimulation and Ask for Social Interaction in an Adolescent with Fragile X Syndrome and Developmental Disabilities** 133	
	Fabrizio Stasolla, Donatella Ciarmoli and Vincenza Albano	
Chapter 7	**Promoting Functional Occupation in a Child with Fragile X Syndrome: Effects on Positive Mood** 147	
	Fabrizio Stasolla, Vincenza Albano and Donatella Ciarmoli	

About the Editor 159

Index 161

PREFACE

Fragile X syndrome is a rare genetic disease caused by mutation of the FMR1 gene located on the X chromosome. It is characterized by mild to moderate or severe to profound developmental disabilities. Phenotype usually includes a long and narrow face, large ears, high-arched palate, flat feet, hyper-extensible finger joints, and large testicles. Typically, it is due to an excessive length (i.e., expansion) of the CGG triplet repeat with fragile X mental retardation 1 gene mutation. Autism-like features are frequently observed. Thus, difficulties in social interactions, delayed speech, aggression, hyperactivity, and seizures are commonly embedded. It is an X-linked dominant inherited disease. Behavioral features may refer to stereotypic movements (i.e., hand-related stereotypy such as biting, flapping, or mouthing), limited eye contact, memory difficulties, shyness, and problems with face encoding. Executive functions, specifically working memory, are significantly compromised. Ataxia, mood disorder, and obsessive-compulsive disorders are additionally acknowledged.

Although no cure exists, early intervention is highly recommended. It provides the most interesting and promising opportunities for acquiring and enhancing a full range of skills. Interventions typically include special education, speech therapy, physical therapy, and behavioral or cognitive-behavioral therapy, next to medication and/or pharmacological treatments related to epilepsy, mood disorders, and/or aggression. Diagnosis is based on DNA results and laboratory or genetic tests. The syndrome is more frequently observed in males who are largely described with full mutation and pre-mutation of the FMR1 gene (i.e., mosaic). Recently, assistive technology-based interventions have been used to improve independence, self-determination, and quality of life among individuals with Fragile X syndrome and to reduce families', caregivers', and professionals' burden accordingly. The book is the result of two decades of professional experience in the field of rehabilitative programs acquired by the editor to promote independence in individuals with multiple disabilities and includes seven chapters.

Chapter One (Rosales-Reynoso, Saucedo-Sariñana, Pérez-Coria, & Barros-Núñez) describes the molecular basis and the pathological mechanisms observed in Fragile X syndrome. A comprehensive literature review was completed using major scientific and bibliographic resources. Data suggested the most interesting advances in the pathological mechanisms of Fragile X and the molecular and sub-cellular dynamics of FMRP (i.e., FMR protein). FMRP was recognized as having a role in the synapses, modulating the local translation of many synaptic proteins whose synthesis is essential for the normal development, maintenance and regulation of dendrites. Among the hundreds of FMRP target mRNAs, only a few have been validated through protein expression or function.

Chapter Two (Tonarelli & Akhter) details the neuropsychiatric symptoms commonly associated with Fragile X syndrome. A critical review of the literature was conducted to summarize the neuropsychiatric disorders seen in patients with FXS. Results evidenced that Fragile X Syndrome is commonly associated with intellectual disability, autism spectrum disorder, several types of anxiety, and attention deficit hyperactivity disorder. Additionally, learning disorders, seizures, and language function disorders are also frequently observed. Obsessive compulsive disorder, mood swings, impulse control behavior, and stereotypies like hand flapping or biting are not unusual. Some individuals have cognitive deficits in the areas of short-term and working memory, visuospatial and mathematic abilities, and executive functions. Rarely, patients can present with catatonia and psychosis. Multiple neuropsychiatric co-morbidities can be presented in cluster in the same patient. FXS is frequently associated with learning disabilities, attention deficit hyperactivity disorder, and epilepsy. Disorders of anxiety and social withdrawal are the core features of the FXS phenotype. The behavioral presentations range from aggression, stereotypies and self-injury behaviors. The clinical presentation of FXS is heterogeneous with clear variation depending on age, gender, and partial or full mutation. Screening for neuropsychiatric disorders is highly recommended to target the specific treatment of the several comorbidities.

Chapter Three (Salcedo-Arellano, Aishworiya, Hagerman, & Protic) argues on pharmacotherapy of Fragile X syndrome. A review of the literature available on pharmacotherapy backed by scientific evidence to support the treatment of psychiatric comorbidities associated with FXS as well as targeted treatments in FXS was proposed. Data presented here were identified by literature searching. Original and review articles, case reports and textbooks in English were used. The source of literature was MEDLINE (1990-2021). The available medications, including mechanism of action, pediatric dosage, target behavior and common adverse effects are compiled. These medications are available clinically and have proven to be beneficial to treat challenging behaviors and common mood disorders affecting individuals with FXS. Off-label targeted treatments are promising for the improvement of various cognitive functions, language development and dysregulated behavior.

Chapter Four (Ciarmoli & Stasolla) summarizes the general features and conceptual issues of Fragile X syndrome. Some relevant issues were addressed. Specifically, molecular and genetic features, brain structure, intellectual development, social communication, challenging behavior, pharmacological intervention, and cognitive-behavioral interventions were discussed. A comprehensive review of the related concerns was outlined. Specific combined interventions were warranted.

Chapter Five (Ciarmoli & Stasolla) evidences a case report. A microswitch-cluster technology was used in two boys with Fragile X syndrome to promote object manipulation and reduce mouthing. Results demonstrate that the technology is useful to pursue the dual simultaneous goal in a unique rehabilitative, technology-based, intervention.

Chapter Six (Stasolla, Ciarmoli, & Albano) describes the implementation of a combined intervention of microswitch and VOCA to enable an adolescent with Fragile X syndrome and severe to profound developmental delays with independent access to positive stimulation and the ability to ask for social interactions with his parents. The intervention was helpful to encourage the participant in positive participation. Thus, he profitably learned the functional use of both technological supports and improved his active role and constructive engagement accordingly. Finally, the adolescent was ensured with the opportunity of choice (between both aforementioned options).

Chapter Seven (Stasolla, Albano, & Ciarmoli) evaluates the use of an assistive technology-based program to provide a boy diagnosed with Fragile X with the awareness of choice. A functional task (i.e., sorting objects in three containers) was proposed. Different environmental consequences were automatically delivered contingently. Data showed that the participant performed the functional task correctly and evidenced the acquired awareness of choice among the environmental consequences, which were systematically and randomly inverted whenever associated to the containers' positions.

The volume highlights useful insights to clinicians, researchers, parents of individuals with Fragile X syndrome, caregivers, and teachers who cope with such pathology in everyday life settings and conditions. Some useful tips may be acknowledged along the different contributions included in the volume.

Fabrizio Stasolla

In: Fragile X Syndrome
Editor: Fabrizio Stasolla

ISBN: 978-1-68507-572-9
© 2022 Nova Science Publishers, Inc.

Chapter 1

FRAGILE X SYNDROME: PATHOLOGICAL MECHANISMS AND MOLECULAR BASES

Mónica Alejandra Rosales-Reynoso[1,*],
Anilú Margarita Saucedo-Sariñana[1],
Mariana Pérez-Coria[1] *and Patricio Barros-Núñez*[2]

[1]División de Medicina Molecular, Centro de Investigación Biomédica de Occidente, CMNO, IMSS, Guadalajara, Jalisco, México
[2]Unidad de Investigación Seguimiento Enfermedades Metabólicas, UMAE Pediatría, CMNO, IMSS, Guadalajara, Jalisco, México

ABSTRACT

Background

Fragile X syndrome (FXS) is the most common inherited cause of intellectual disability. FXS occurs in the absence of fragile X mental retardation protein 1 (FMRP), which is a regulator of synaptic and postsynaptic mRNAs. The FMRP absence is caused by a greater than 200

---

[*] Corresponding Author's E-mails: mareynoso77@yahoo.com.mx; monica.rosales@imss.gob.mx.

CGG repeats expansion in the promoter region of the *FMR1* gene, which induces its hypermethylation, inactivation, and the characteristic clinical picture. Expansions of 55 to 200 repeats are named premutations and increase mRNA expression that in adults is associated with the tremor/ataxia phenotype and primary ovarian failure. Diagnosis is traditionally made by detecting CGG expansion by PCR or Southern Blot analysis. Different studies have clarified that brain alterations underlying clinical manifestations are related to neuronal plasticity, GABAergic activity, and increased translation of different proteins.

Objectives

This chapter aims to review current developments on the pathological mechanisms as well as the molecular bases of the disease that allow a better understanding of the FXS mutated and premutated allele phenotypes.

Method

A comprehensive literature review was completed using major scientific and bibliographic resources.

Results

A coherent and up-to-date summary of this review is presented on the most interesting advances in the pathological mechanisms of fragile X and the molecular and subcellular dynamics of FMRP.

Conclusion

FMRP plays an essential role in the synapses, modulating the local translation of many synaptic proteins whose synthesis is essential for the normal development, maintenance, and regulation of dendrites. Among the hundreds of FMRP target mRNAs, only a few have been validated through the protein expression or function.

Keywords: Fragile X syndrome, *FMR1*, intellectual disability, CGG repeats, permutated phenotypes, FMRP, treatment

1. INTRODUCTION

Intellectual disability (ID) is caused by a highly heterogeneous number of causes, ranging from genetic to environmental or a combination of both [1, 2]. The Fragile X Syndrome (FXS), caused by silencing of the expression of Fragile X Mental Retardation gene 1 (*FMR1*), is the most common monogenic source of inherited ID, affecting 1/4000 males and 1/7000 females [3–5]. In males, this condition is characterized by moderate to severe intellectual affectation, whereas 60% of carrier females present only mild to moderate disability [4, 5]. The *FMR1* gene encodes a protein (FMRP) involved in the RNA post-transcriptional regulation with essential roles in synaptic plasticity, in the development of dendrites and axons, and underlying learning and memory [4].

FXS affected individuals are characterized by hyperactive and/or autistic behavior, attention deficit, sleep disorders, epileptic seizures, facial dysmorphism, connective tissue dysplasia, and post-pubertal macroorchidism [1]. Histopathological examination of the brain shows an increased density of long dendritic spines, considered the main subcellular defect in both FXS animal models and FXS patients [4]. Silencing of the expression of the *FMR1* gene and consequent lack of FMRP in most FXS patients is caused by a large trinucleotide CGG-repeat expansion in the untranslated region 5´-UTR of the gene, resulting in transcriptional inactivation of the *FMR1* gene. Only rare cases have been reported carrying a partially deleted or mutated *FMR1* gene [3–5].

Numerous molecular and functional studies have characterized the general and subcellular dynamics of FMRP. In brief, FMRP enters the nucleus and interacts with pre-messenger ribonucleoprotein (pre-mRNP) complexes to guide them to the cytoplasm. FMRP-containing mRNPs are then associated with polyribosomes and involved in translational control both in the soma and in distant pre and post-synaptic regions [6]. RNA-binding proteins (RBPs) recognize and bind mRNA to targets in the coding regions and also to 5' and 3' untranslated regions (UTRs) [7]. Several RBPs cooperate and increase the specificity of this interaction. The actin cytoskeleton facilitates RNA recognition, as this structure associates with

RBPs [8]. Individual RBPs bind to several mRNAs, which has led to a model of regulated gene expression in eukaryotes, termed "the post-transcriptional operon" [9]. FMRP is a widely studied RBP in the brain, the absence of which leads to FXS [5].

In subcellular sites, there is a well-known mechanism of protein synthesis that enables the rapid expression of specific genes in particular regions as a response to localized signals [10]. During the transport of mRNA to these regions, it is stabilized by numerous and different factors, such as RNA-binding proteins (RBPs) and non-coding RNAs, forming ribonucleic particles (RNPs) that vary in composition and size during the cell cycle or the development. In polarized cells as neurons, mRNAs are transported from the nucleus to dendrites and axons, where these molecules undergo local translation and degradation [11–13].

In neurons, FMRP-mRNP complexes are selectively transported to distant locations as a component of RNA-granules, by binding mRNAs and molecular motors such as kinesins, promoting transport upon specific stimuli. Reduced capacity to transport and translate mRNA into distal processes results in an abnormal level of their protein products, with variable consequences on different subcellular structures, as observed in animal models and FXS patients [14]. The mutational mechanism of the *FMR1* gene observed in the FXS has also been associated with the pathogenesis of other disorders, such as premature ovarian failure (POF), fragile X-associated tremor ataxia syndrome (FXTAS), and autism spectrum disorder (ASD) [5].

This chapter aims to review the current development on pathological mechanisms, as well as the molecular bases of this disease, in order to understand the phenotypes resulting from the mutated and premutated alleles of the *FMR1* gene, as well as their treatment possibilities.

2. Fragile X Syndrome (#MIM 300624)

FXS is the most common cause (1-2%) of inherited intellectual disability (ID) and the leading form of monogenic autism and autistic spectrum disorders (ASD) [15, 16]. The *FMR1* gene is inherited as an X-linked dominant trait with reduced penetrance of 80% in males and 30-50% in females; however, due to X-inactivation in females and genetic anticipation, the inheritance of FXS does not follow standard X-linked dominant inheritance. Females with the full *FMR1* mutation exhibit a milder phenotype, as a result of the variation in the X-inactivation [17]. The *FMR1* gene encodes for a protein (FMRP) which is involved in the RNA post-transcriptional regulation and plays an important role in synaptic plasticity, in the development of dendrites and axons, and underlying learning and memory [17, 18].

The great majority of FXS patients show a lack of FMRP due to a large trinucleotide CGG-repeat expansion of the first exon of the *FMR1* gene. The consequent hypermethylation of the CGG repeats and adjacent CpG islands cause the *FMR1* gene silencing [9]. Rare cases have been reported carrying a partially deleted or mutated *FMR1* gene [17]. Therefore, the methylation status of CGG triplets is a key factor for classifying FXS; the greater the degree of methylation, the greater the deficit of FMRP. A molecular consequence of reduced FMRP is the hyperactivation of the extracellular-signal-regulated kinase (ERK) signaling pathway and the mammalian target of rapamycin complex 1 (mTORC1) [17].

The number of CGG repeats is polymorphic between normal populations and varies from 6 to 44 [19, 20]; the adjacent CpG islands, which act as a promoter, are non-methylated and remain stable upon transmission. The second class of alleles within the upper-normal range contains 45 to 54 CGGs. This range is known as the "gray zone" and corresponds to intermediate alleles that can be slightly unstable and transmitted to successive generations with the possibility of expanding to a premutated or intermediate allele [21].

The frequency of premutated alleles (55 to 200 CGGs) varies in the general population from 1/35 to 1/57 [22]. In premutated alleles, the CpG islands are non-methylated and the *FMR1* gene is transcribed and translated; however, premutation carriers show normal or slightly reduced synthesis of FMRP with increased levels of mRNA (2-8-fold more than normal alleles) and are asymptomatic for FXS. Premutation carriers have an increased risk of affected offspring because the number of CGGs is unstable and tends to increase with each cellular division. Moreover, people carrying premutation alleles are at risk of developing some disorders as Fragile X-associated tremor/ataxia syndrome (FXTAS) and Fragile X premature ovarian insufficiency (FXPOI), and emotional disorders, among others [22] (Figure 1).

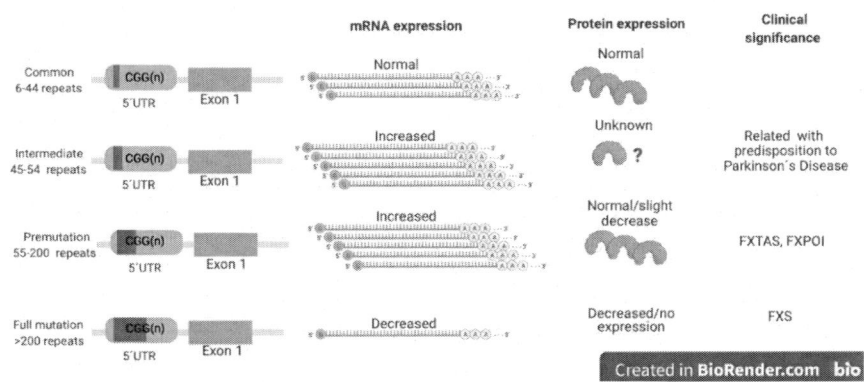

Figure 1. The type of *FMR1* alleles, its mRNA and FMRP expression with their clinical implications are characterized. The normal alleles contain 6-44 CGG repeats. The intermediate alleles contain 45-54 CGG repeats with increased expression of mRNA, unknown FMRP expression and related to Parkinson´s disease. The premutated alleles contain 55-200 CGG repeats; its mRNA expression is increased with normal to slightly decreased FMRP and is related to Fragile X-associated tremor/ataxia syndrome (FXTAS) and Fragile X premature ovarian insufficiency (FXPOI). The full mutated alleles contain >200 CGG repeats, which leads to increase methylation of the *FMR1* gene and decreased or null production of mRNA and FMRP, resulting in the Fragile X syndrome phenotype [31].

2.1. Clinical Features

Clinical manifestations of classic FXS have not important variations since its first description; in boys with FXS, the physical characteristics include a long face, large and prominent ears, postpubertal macroorchidism, and hyperextensible joints. Additional features include velvet-like skin, a high-arched palate, flat feet, pectus excavatum, connective tissue dysplasia, and cardiac abnormalities with subsequence mitral valve prolapse [23–26]. The frequency of FXS is variable according to the population; however, 1/4,000 men and 1/7,000 women is an acceptable number worldwide [27]. The most important functional and psychological features in FXS are shown in Table 1-A.

2.2. Historical Aspects

Although 80 years have passed since the first description by Martin and Bell (1943), there is still much to discern about this condition. It took about 20 years to add other clinical observations in these patients, and it was not until 1969 that fragile sites were observed, specifically at the terminal end of the long arm of the X chromosome (Xq27.3) giving rise to the name of "Fragile X syndrome" [2]. In 1991, 3 groups independently cloned the *FMR1* gene. Later in the 80´s, it was reported that certain folate antagonist drugs increase the risk of FXS in pregnant women. In addition, other authors considered theories about a possible genetic modifier that would explain why healthy intellectually women had children affected with FXS [3–5]. Figure 2 shows a timeline with the main findings related to FXS.

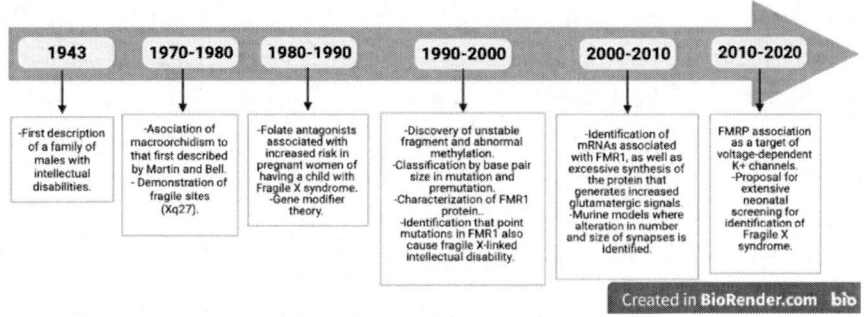

Figure 2. Timeline of the main FXS findings.

2.3. Premutated Allele Phenotypes

The *FMR1* gene and the FMRP have also been associated with the pathogenesis of other disorders, such as Fragile X-associated tremor ataxia syndrome (FXTAS) and Fragile X premature ovarian insufficiency (FXPOI) [15].

2.3.1. *FXS Associated with Tremor Ataxia Syndrome (FXTAS)*

FXTAS is observed in 70% of men carrying the *FMR1* premutation (55-200 CGG repeats) over 70 years old; however, only 16% of women carriers of premutation developing FXTAS [28, 29]. The clinical presentation consists of intention tremor, gait ataxia, progressive neurodegeneration, Parkinsonism, cognitive decline, and white matter abnormalities observed in magnetic resonance imaging (MRI). The main functional and psychological features observed in FXTAS patients are summarized in Table 1-B. To understand the pathophysiology of FXTAS, animal models as mouse and *Drosophila melanogaster* have been implemented; these models exhibit overexpression of *FMR1* mRNA and lower expression of FMRP protein, intranuclear inclusions, and other common characteristics of FXTAS as abnormal dendritic spine morphology, impaired coordination and cognitive deficits [29].

The molecular mechanisms implied in the pathophysiology of FXTAS are mRNA-gain and repeated-associated non-ATG (RAN) translation [30]. The overexpression of *FMR1* mRNA generates aggregates of CGG binding proteins; however, in the intranuclear inclusions, some proteins do not have interactions with CGG sites. On the other hand, the RAN translation of 5´ UTR of *FMR1* mRNA produces toxic peptides with polyglycine (FMR-polyG) [29]. There is no specific treatment for this syndrome, but some medications are used for the psychiatric issues and tremor severity [28].

2.3.2. FXS Associated Primary Ovarian Insufficiency (FXPOI)

Females carrying a premutation in the *FMR1* gene can develop primary ovarian insufficiency in adulthood, with diminished ovarian reserve, menstrual cycle irregularities, hormonal fluctuations, decreased fertility, and early menopause (before 40 years old) [31]. The main functional and psychological features in FXPOI patients are summarized in Table 1-C.

To date, there is not a molecular mechanism that can explain clearly how this happens, but some animal models have been studied. *Drosophila melanogaster* with mutated *FMR1* has fewer eggs, which confirms that FMRP is necessary to the maintenance of germline stem cells [32]. In humans, the FMRP is expressed in germ cells surrounded by FMRP-negative pregranulose and interstitial cells, and its expression coincides with a loss of expression of the pluripotency-associated protein. In carriers with premutation of *FMR1*, the reduced expression of FMRP could influence the maintenance of stem cells and dismiss the quantity follicular [32].

Table 1. Functional and psychological features in Fragile X syndrome, FXTAS and FXPOI patients

A) Fragile X syndrome	B) Fragile X-associated tremor and ataxia syndrome (FXTAS)	C) Primary ovarian insufficiency (FXPOI) (Carrier frequency 1:178)
• Infancy: hypotonia, poor suck, mild motor delay, seizures, language delay. • Early childhood and adolescence: Impulsivity, autism symptoms, anxiety. • Adulthood-Ageing: Anxiety, perseveration, Parkinsonism symptoms [33].	• Intention tremor, cerebellar ataxia, neuropathic pain, memory and/or executive function deficit, Parkinsonism, and psychological disorders. • Brain atrophy and white matter disease (middle cerebellar peduncles) [34].	• Menstrual dysfunction, early menopause, infertility. • Anxiety, major depressive disorder, sleep disturbances • Thyroid dysfunction • Cardiovascular morbidity • Neuropathy, fibromyalgia [35].

3. FMRP STRUCTURE

3.1. The *FMR1* Gene and Its Protein Product

The human *FMR1* gene was cloned in 1991 [36]; located at the cytogenetic position Xq27.3, contains 17 exons spanning 38 kb [37, 38]. The *FMR1* gene suffers alternative splicing in exons 12, 14, 15 and 17, resulting in several *FMR1* mRNA isoforms [39]. The distribution of these isoforms differs according to the different brain areas [38]. FMRP contains several functional domains: two K-homology motifs (KH1 and KH2), a RGG box, a nuclear localization signal (NLS), and a nuclear export signal (NES). In addition, there is also evidence that the N- terminus has an RNA-binding activity [40, 41] (Figure 3).

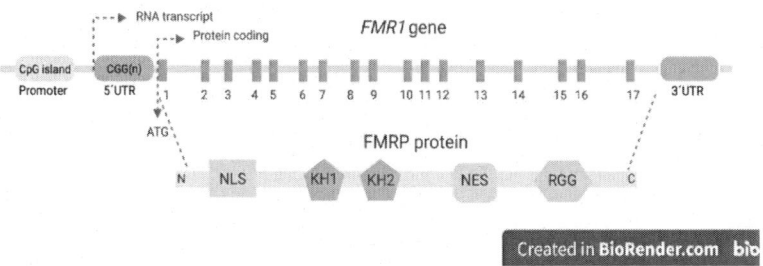

Figure 3. The *FMR1* gene consists of 17 exons and codes to the FMRP protein. The gene has a CpG island in the promoter region, and the 5´ UTR region contains a variable region with repeats CGG(n). The FMRP protein has five domains: nuclear localization signal (NLS), KH1 y KH2 domains, the nuclear export signal (NES) and the motif glycine-arginine rich (RGG) [31].

FMRP is a highly conserved multifunctional RNA binding protein, mainly expressed in testes and the brain, and plays a significant role in synaptic plasticity [12, 31, 42, 43]. FMRP expression has also been observed in epithelial tissues, respiratory epithelium, small intestine, stomach, large bowel, and esophagus [44]. Within the brain, the most intense location occurs in neuron-rich regions, including the cerebellum and hypothalamus, with a clear signal seen principally in the cell body of the neurons [44, 45]. Cells of the white matter, including oligodendrocytes and astrocytes, likely contain very little FMRP [45]. In mammal's brains, FMRP binds to approximately 4% of mRNAs to regulate protein synthesis. The lack of FMRP implies additional basal translation [46].

RNA-binding domains of FMRP mediate FMRP-RNA interactions: the mRNA G quartet that binds to the RGG box, and the mRNA named "kissing complex" that binds to the KH2 domain [47]. Novel RNA structural motifs recognized by FMRP include Sod1 mRNA Stem Loops interacting (SoSLIP) within the mRNA for superoxide dismutase (SOD1), which increases the translation of SOD1 mRNA as a positive modulator role of FMRP [48].

It has been described that FMRP can also regulate translation by actively binding to translating polyribosomes in an RNA-dependent interaction in non-neural and neural cell lines [49]. The KH domains seem to be important for this translational control [50]. The importance of the RNA-binding function of FMRP is further emphasized by the observation that an *FMR1* gene point mutation (I304N), alters RNA binding to polyribosome and leads to a severe neurological phenotype of FXS [51, 52]. One-third of all RNAs encoding pre-and postsynaptic proteins are targets of FMRP. This role as a transcription factor may explain the phenotypic complexity of the FXS and its variable expression [16]. In the mammalian brain, FMRP targets hundreds of coding and non-coding RNAs, and a few microRNAs [41, 53–56]. Later its homodimerization, FMRP interacts with numerous cytoplasmic and nuclear proteins that participate in cytoskeleton-remodeling and mRNA metabolism [15]. The FMRP Ile304Asn mutation reduces the binding affinity to numerous mRNAs, such as *FMR1*, bifunctional glutamate/proline-tRNA ligase (EPRS), neurofibromatosis type 1 (NF1), structural maintenance of chromosomes protein 1A (SMC1A), serine/threonine-protein phosphatase 2A catalytic subunit alpha isoform (PPP2CA), ubiquitin-protein ligase E3A (UBE3A), and cohesin subunit SA-2 (STAG2) [57].

4. FMRP FUNCTION

FMRP is the major RNA binding protein that inhibits the translation of RNA targets; mainly in the spermatogonia and brain, it is constitutively expressed from the early stages of development until postnatal life [58]. The localization of the FMRP is mainly cytoplasmatic, associated with the polyribosomes attached to the endoplasmic reticulum and with free ribosomes at the bases of dendrites and within dendritic spines [59]. FMRP plays an essential role in the synapses; in healthy neurons, FMRP modulates the local translation of several synaptic proteins whose synthesis is essential for the normal development, maintenance, and regulation of dendrites [56].

4.1. Stability of mRNA

Some studies performed in Fmr1 KO mice reveal that the absence of FMRP alters hundreds of mRNAs in the brain [60]. FMRP modulates the stability of some mRNAs by preventing or sustaining mRNA decay [61]. As an example, the hippocampal FMRP protects PSD-95 mRNA from decay in an activity-dependent manner; however, FMRP also facilitates the decay of nuclear RNA export factor 1 (NXF1) mRNA in mouse neuroblastoma (N2a) cells [62, 63].

4.2. Transport of mRNA

FMRP granules transport RNA/mRNAs (including its own) from the cell body to synapses by association with microtubule motors in an activity-dependent manner [64–66]. Furthermore, FMRP regulates translation at cortical synapses [67]. The cortical region of the Fmr1 KO mouse brain shows the reduced expression of different GABA A receptor subunits [60], consistent with imbalanced GABAergic signaling in FXS patients.

4.3. Translation of mRNA

Studies performed in lymphoblastoid cells derived from FXS individuals showed an augmented translation rate in several FMRP targets [11]. Increased translation of FMRP mRNA targets was also observed in Fmr1 KO mice, specifically at synapses, consistent with the idea that FMRP functions as a repressor of translation [11, 67, 68]. FMRP activity is regulated in response to different signaling cascades, i.e., the 2-amino-3-(5-methyl-3-oxo-1,2-oxazol-4-yl) propanoic acid (AMPA) receptors, type I metabotropic glutamate receptors (mGluRs), the N-methyl-D-aspartate (NMDA) receptors, the γ-aminobutyric acid (GABA) receptors, the dopamine (DA) receptors, the tyrosine kinase or BDNF/NT-3 growth factor (TrkB) receptors, and recently the cannabinoid receptors [69].

One of the most affected and well-characterized signaling cascades in FXS is the mGluR [70]. Once activated the mGluR receptor, FMRP-mediated translational block is released, and protein synthesis occurs. In the absence of FMRP, the increase in protein synthesis results in a receptor imbalance; an increase in the mGluR1 and mGluR5 activity and the reduced insertion of AMPA receptors at the surface leads to enhanced mGluR long-term depression (mGluR-LTD), that involves mRNA targeting and local protein synthesis and degradation, which can be induced through the application of (S)-3,5-dihydroxyphenylglycine (DHPG) in a protein synthesis-independent manner [12]. In Fmr1 KO mice, DHPG-induced LTD is increased, and these electrophysiological phenotypes established the "mGluR theory" in FXS [33, 70].

FMRP activity is controlled through posttranslational modifications. DHPG-induced LTD also activates FMRP synthesis at synapses [10, 65, 71], which in turn is rapidly degraded through the ubiquitin-proteasome system [72]. The effect of FMRP on protein synthesis is influenced by phosphorylation of FMRP through the mTOR signaling pathway [73, 74].

FMRP has also been detected in stress granules (SG), P bodies (PB), and cytoplasmic structures containing translationally silent pre-initiation complexes [75]. FMRP represses translation through its binding to CYFIP1, a neuronal eIF4E-BP. CYFIP1 binds to eIF4E, blocking the initiation of translation. Consequently, the synaptic stimuli CYFIP1-FMRP complex is released from eIF4E and translation ensues [76]. In addition, FMRP has also been proposed to regulate mRNA elongation [33, 58].

4.4. A Potential Nuclear Function of FMRP

FMRP is mostly found in the cytoplasm, but evidence supports a potential nuclear function. The NES and NLS domains of FMRP are responsible for the shuttling of the protein between the cytoplasm and nucleus. Moreover, FMRP is involved in mRNA transport and nuclear export of m6-A-containing mRNAs [77] and in the replication-stress-induced DNA damage response [78]. FMRP isoforms that miss exon 14 lose the NES domain and therefore are retained in the nucleus [79]. The exact function of these isoforms has not yet been elucidated.

5. FXS MOLECULAR PATHOPHYSIOLOGY

FMRP is an RNA binding protein with a role in the translational control of several mRNAs in the postsynaptic compartment of neurons, linked to the activation status of the group 1 metabotropic glutamate receptor (mGluRI) [80, 81]. Other proposed cellular functions include activation of the potassium channels KCNT1 and BK, a chromatin-dependent role in the DNA damage response, and a role in the RNA editing [82–84]. FMRP can also regulate neuronal activity, including hippocampal-dependent learning and the endocannabinoid system [85, 86]. In addition, it has been involved in the BMPR2-cofilin pathway [33].

5.1. Glutamatergic Signaling

Increased glutamate signaling probably underlies several of the clinical manifestations of FXS. Long-term depression dependent on metabotropic glutamate receptor 1 (mGluRI-LTD) is increased in the hippocampus [33, 12] and the cerebellum of Fmr1-knockout mice [87]. Pharmacological block of these receptors corrected the phenotype of the Fmr1-knockout mouse, including seizures, hyperactivity, and neuronal structural changes, demonstrating excessive mGluRI signaling [46] and emphasized mGluRI antagonists as a potential treatment for FXS [33, 88, 89].

The main consequence of mGluRI activation is the translation of postsynaptic proteins involved in synaptic plasticity potentiation; specifically, mGluRI-LTD, by remodeling the protein content of dendritic spines [33, 90, 91]. Elevated phosphorylation of S6K likely causes the excessive protein synthesis of FMRP-target mRNAs observed in vivo and in vitro in several areas of the Fmr1knockout mouse brain, notably in hippocampal and cortical neurons [92, 93]. This increased protein synthesis seems to be of crucial importance for the pathophysiology of FXS, as several inhibitors of translation have rescuing effects on the mouse phenotypes [33, 80, 81].

On the other hand, several methods have been used to identify which gene products are altered in absence of FMRP. Among the hundreds of FMRP target mRNAs, only a few have been validated through the protein expression or function. The deregulated proteins with a possibly more-prominent role in the pathophysiology of FXS include phosphatidylinositol 3 kinase enhancer (PIKE), $GABA_A$ and $GABA_B$ receptor subunits [33, 94, 95], matrix metalloproteinase 9 (MMP9) [96], glycogen synthase kinase 3 (GSK3) [97], amyloid-β A4 protein (APP) [98] and diacylglycerol kinase-κ (DGKκ) [99]. The inhibition of PIKE, GSK3, and APP expression in FXS might be helpful treatments but has not yet been evaluated in human studies [33, 98, 100].

FMRP is also associated with MMP9 mRNA, which encodes an endopeptidase crucial for dendritic spine maturation [101]. MMP9 levels are increased in FXS but can be lowered to normal levels with minocycline treatment [102]. In Fmr1-knockout mice, treatment with minocycline improves synapse formation, dendritic spine maturation, anxiety levels, and cognitive performance [103]. Remarkably, metformin can also lower MMP9 levels in the Fmr1-knockout mouse [104].

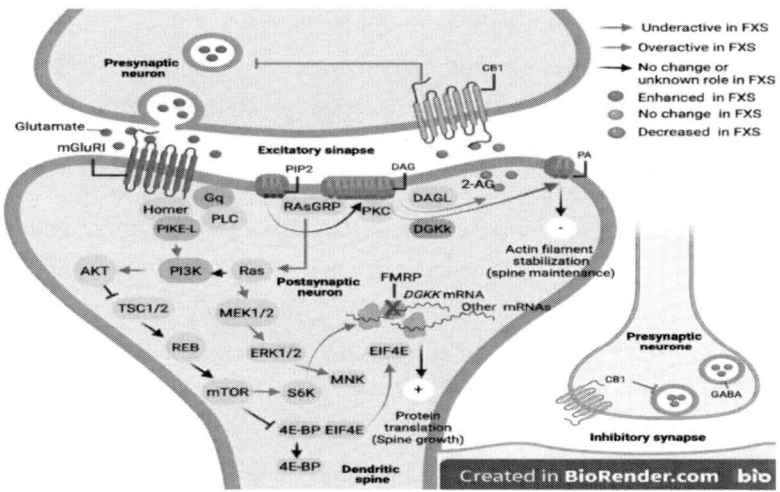

Figure 4. Glutamatergic pathway. The signaling of the mGluRI receptor activates the production of Diacylglycerol (DAG), the protein kinase C (PKC), the phosphoinositide 3-kinase (PI3K)-AKT-mTOR and the ERK pathway. The DAG is converted to 2-arachidonylglycerol (2-AG), this inhibits the release of glutamate and aminobutyric acid (GABA) via cannabinoid type 1 receptor (CB1). In absence of FMRP, there is an overactivation of PKC, PI3K-AKT-mTOR and RAS-MEK-ERK. DGKκ phosphorylates DAG to phosphatidic acid (PA), and PA regulates several pathways as RAC-PAK, mTOR and RAF1-kinase. In FXS the expression of DGKk is decreased, this leads to over activation of DAG signaling and results in dendritic spine growth and reduced dendritic stabilization [33].

In cortical neurons, FMRP is largely associated with DGKk mRNA, whose protein converts diacylglycerol (DAG) to phosphatidic acid (PA) [100]. DGKκ is a member of the DGK family (10 isoforms) [105]; only DGKk mRNA can bind to FMRP. DGKs are involved in diverse biological processes as cytokine-dependent cell proliferation, seizure activity, motility, immune responses, glucose metabolism, and cardiovascular responses [106]. Accordingly, DGK proteins are involved in several diseases, such as epilepsy, bipolar disorder, Parkinson's disease, hypertension, cardiac hypertrophy, type 2 diabetes mellitus, autoimmunity, and cancer. DGKκ expression is decreased in the Fmr1-knockout mouse, which causes an imbalance of DAG and PA levels, with consequent dendritic spine growth and stabilization (Figure 4) [99, 107]. Reduction of DGKκ expression in the mouse striatum by short hairpin RNA caused autistic behavior, similar to those observed in the Fmr1-knockout mouse; reversely, overexpression of DGKκ rescued the impaired dendritic spine morphology [33, 99]. FMRP would control the protein translation within dendritic spines by an indirect (DAG-mediated) rather than a direct (RNA-binding) mechanism [33, 99].

5.2. Endocannabinoid System

The lack of FMRP also alters the endocannabinoid system through their receptors located in peripheral nerves and the brain, which are involved in various processes as cognitive performance, synaptic plasticity, nociception, seizure susceptibility, and anxiety. The endocannabinoid ligands bind to the G protein-coupled receptors CB1 and CB2 and modulate synaptic activity [33, 108, 109]. 2-AG is the most abundant endocannabinoid ligand in the brain and is produced locally within dendritic spines following mGluRI activation (Figure 4). In the FXS mouse, endogenous stimulation of 2-AG receptors leads to synaptic plasticity abnormalities, including enhanced LTD at inhibitory synapses [110–112] and decreased LTD at excitatory synapses [113]. Inhibiting 2-AG degradation [113] or blocking CB1 and CB2 receptors [112] can normalize some alterations in the FXS mouse [33].

5.3. GABAergic System

Alterations in GABAergic signaling have been detected in the brains of Fmr1-knockout mice, including a reduction in the expression of several

GABA receptor subunits (Figure 5). Electrophysiological studies have demonstrated that GABA$_A$ receptor-mediated signaling is compromised in the Fmr1-knockout mouse [33, 114–117]; specifically, defects in phasic (synaptic) and tonic (extrasynaptic) inhibitory signaling and a delay in the transition from excitatory to inhibitory GABAergic signaling during development [33, 118].

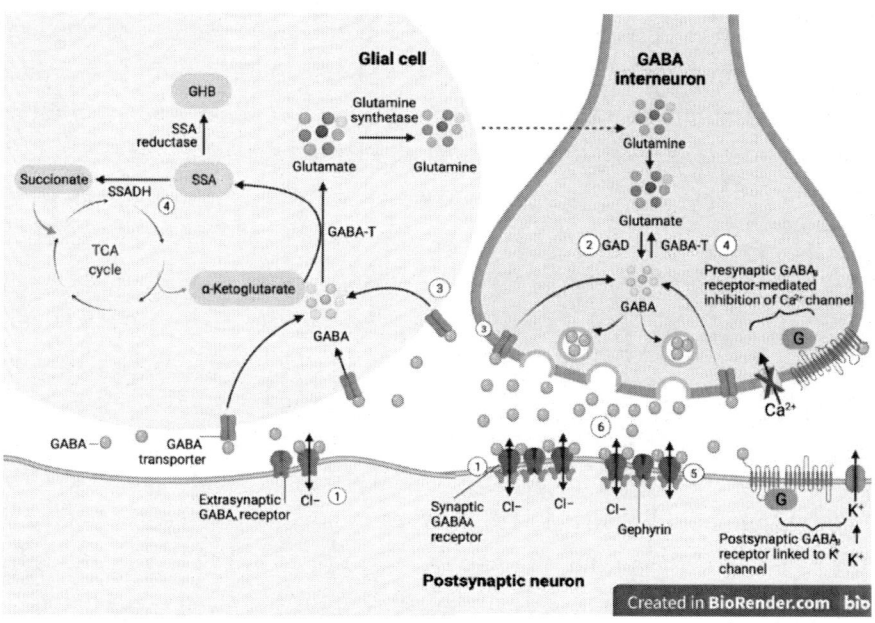

Figure 5. GABAergic signalling in *Fmr1* knockout mice. In the postsynaptic neuron, the gamma aminobutyric acid A receptor (GABA$_A$) is integrated for several subunits; the protein FMRP participate in the translations of mRNAs of these subunits and in FXS there is a decrease in the half of the subunits ①. On the presynaptic side, FMRP is also expressed, and its absence affects the expression of genes that encoding proteins that participate in the GABA synthesis (*Gad1*, and *Gad2*) which encode glutamate D carboxylase (GAD) ②, GABA transporters ③ and *ABAT* that encodes 4-aminobutyrate aminotransferase (GABA-T) ④, in receptor clustering (*Gphn* encoding gephyrin) ⑤ and GABA free is reduced in Fmr1- knockout mice ⑥ [33].

Preclinical studies in animal models confirmed that the GABA$_A$ receptor is a suitable target [88, 119]. Nine compounds that corrected specific phenotypes in Fmr1deficient Drosophila were identified [120]; of these, three can restore GABA homeostasis. Gaboxadol (also known as THIP), a superagonist of δ-subunit-containing $GABA_A$ receptors, can rescue hyperexcitability of principal neurons of the amygdala of Fmr1-knockout mice and can improve some specific behavioral characteristics, including hyperactivity and auditory seizures [33, 115]. Synthetic neurosteroids such as ganaxolone are potent agonists of $GABA_A$ receptors [121] and can prevent audiogenic seizures and correct repetitive and/or perseverative behaviors in the Fmr1-knockout mouse [122]. Prenatal treatment of Fmr1 knockout mice with bumetanide restored electrophysiological abnormalities in the mutant offspring as well as hyperactivity and autistic behaviors [123].

6. FMRP AND MATRIX METALLOPROTEINASES

Matrix metalloproteinases (MMPs) regulate pathological remodeling processes. MMP-9, one of the most widely investigated MMPs, directly degrades extracellular matrix proteins and activates cytokines and chemokines to regulate tissue remodeling. MMP-9 has a pivotal role in the process of endochondral ossification and skeletal development [124]. Analysis *in silico* of murine MMP-9 revealed that RNA motifs are typically bound by FMRP [125, 126]. Investigating murine hippocampal regions and using RNA co-immunoprecipitation techniques, a complex of MMP-9 mRNA with FMRP was confirmed [125]. Increased MMP-9 protein expression was observed in human FXS post-mortem brain samples and hippocampus of young and adult Fmr1 KO mice [103, 127]. The translation of synaptic MMP-9 is regulated by FMRP in a mouse model; the absence of FMRP in *Fmr1* KO mice increases the MMP-9 mRNA translation at hippocampal synapses [125]. Minocycline, a drug that inhibits MMP-9 activity in FXS animal models, results in mature dendrite formation and improves behavioral deficits; therefore, it can be considered a promising therapeutic option in FXS patients [31, 102, 128, 129].

7. FMRP AND CANCER

FMRP has been involved in cancer progression, metastasis formation, and tumor invasiveness. FMRP is overexpressed in human hepatocellular carcinoma, breast cancer, pancreatic ductal adenocarcinoma, melanoma, and murine neuroendocrine tumors [126, 130–133]. In 2007, Kalkunte et al. found a minimized glioblastoma invasion in a patient diagnosed with FXS [134]. In addition, there is evidence that patients with FXS present a decreased risk of developing cancer [135]. In 2010, Rosales-Reynoso et al. identified *WNT7A* as a gene associated with diminished cancer risk in FXS patients [136]. In contrast, a high level of FMRP is linked to metastatic breast cancer, and overexpression of the protein in primary breast tumors induces lung metastasis [137]. In another study [130], a high level of FMRP expression correlated significantly with metastatic melanoma tissues; meanwhile, a reduction of FMRP in metastatic melanoma cell lines affects cell migration, invasion, and adhesion.

In 2019, Zhu et al. showed that circKSCAN1 suppressed the cell stem in hepatocellular carcinoma by regulating the function of FMRP. They identified the cell cycle and apoptosis regulator 1 (CCAR1) as the downstream target gene of FMRP, which acts as a co-activator of the Wnt/β-catenin signaling pathway and up-regulates cell stemness. The results of that study revealed a novel mechanism whereby circRNAs regulate malignant behavior in cancers, in addition to acting as a miRNA sponge [138]. On the other hand, Van Dijck et al. (2020) found that patients with FXS exhibit reduced serum levels of several chemokines and may therefore exhibit impaired immune responses [139].

Recent studies have shown the participation of FMRP in colorectal cancer (CRC) and hepatocellular carcinoma (HCC) [140, 141]. In 2001, Di Grazia et al., studying human CRC cell lines, demonstrated that FMRP binds to the receptor-interacting protein kinase 1 (RIPK1) mRNA, and suggested that FMRP participate in the necroptosis pathway through regulating the RIPK1 mRNA metabolism [141]. In 2021, Shen et al. proposed that NUFIP1 is overexpressed in CRC and correlates with disease progression and poor survival. NUFIP1 is an RNA-binding protein that interacts with FMRP in the messenger ribonucleoprotein particle (mRNP) and may exert oncogenic effects by altering senescence [140].

On the other hand, Shen et al. 2021 observed that FMRP promotes and modulates the localization and translation of STAT3 mRNA in cell protrusions, accelerating the metastasis in HCC. Serine 114 of FMRP could be a potential phosphorylation site required for IL-6-mediated STAT3 translation. FMRP is highly expressed in HCC tissues, and FMRP knockdown efficiently suppresses HCC metastasis in vitro and in vivo [140].

All these findings demonstrate that overexpression of FMRP can be linked to certain types of cancers. As an RNA binding protein, FMRP binds to several RNA targets while controlling their translation, transport, and stability [142]. FMRP bind to G-quadruplex (G4) motifs on RNA, a structure organized in repeating units of guanine tetrads, through the RGG domain [143, 144]. The G-quadruplex motifs are involved in regulating different steps of RNA metabolism; in particular, FMRP-RNA complexes regulate translation and additional post-transcriptional regulatory functions [143–145]. RNA G4 structures participate in regulating the expression of genes implicated in cancer, including *TP53*, *VEGF*, *hTERT*, *TGFB2*, and other essential oncogenes [146]. These findings support the conclusion that FMRP is overexpressed in specific cancers and plays a significant role in tumor progression through altered FMRP-dependent G4 mRNA expression.

The copper/zinc dismutase *SOD1* is overexpressed in cancers and localized in the cytoplasm, the inter-membrane space of mitochondria, and the nucleus [147]. Through its RGG motif, FMRP recognizes the SoSLIP RNA motif (Sod1 mRNA Stem Loops Interacting with FMRP) and binds Sod1 mRNA with a high affinity to activate its translation [48]. FMRP overexpression and positive regulation of Sod1 translation can directly or indirectly influence cancer progression [145, 147].

8. Treatments for Fragile X Syndrome

Current knowledge of neurobiology and synaptic mechanisms in FXS has generated new opportunities for more efficient treatments for autism and related disorders. FXS represents an outstanding model for understanding and translating the molecular findings to neurologic treatments; interestingly, all affected individuals exhibit the same gene defect causing its clinical condition. A significant number of mechanisms through which the genetic defect modifies the molecular events in neurons and its synaptic process are now extensively known in FXS individuals. As result, several models have been proposed to explain such a crescent number of neurodevelopmental conditions as autistic spectrum disorders (ASDs), learning disability, attention deficit, and hyperactivity disorders (ADHD).

Many studies and intense efforts have been dedicated to finding specific FXS treatments. In resume, two approaches are considered for a probable treatment of FXS: 1) Reactivation of the mutated *FMR1* gene, and 2) Compensation of the lacked FMR1 protein. In this context, the current therapeutic methodologies intend to modulate some chemical-biological systems related to the FMR1 metabolic pathways as mGluR5 antagonists, GABA receptor agonists, GSK3B inhibitors, NMDA antagonists, and other FMRP downstream targets [148-149]. Among the behavioral problems, symptoms to treat are aggression, anxiety, seizures, and attention deficit. The educational stimuli have also been beneficial in facilitating the development of self-care and social and adaptive behaviors. Together, these treatments can raise the quality of life for both patients and their families. Among the most noticeable studies related to clinical treatments targeted to FXS, the group of mGluRs result quite interesting.

8.1. mGluR5 Antagonists

Many excitatory synapses express Group 1 Metabotropic Glutamate Receptors (Gp1 mGluRs) at the synaptic periphery [148]. Activation of mGluRs usually occurs in response to intense activity and triggers long-term plasticity of synaptic transmission in many brain regions including the neocortex, hippocampus, midbrain, striatum, and cerebellum [33]. Gp1 mGluRs (1 and 5) induce both long-term depression (LTD) and potentiation (LTP) of synaptic strength. Among the mGluRs antagonists, mGluR5 is highly interesting given its activity in the neocortex, hippocampus, and striatum [148]. As other G-protein coupled, the mGluRs transduce excitatory signals via 1. Phosphoinositol (PI) and phospholipase C (PLC), 2. Phosphoinositide in the PI3K/AKT/mTOR cascade, and 3. Extracellular signal-regulated kinase (ERK) cascade [148]. In the absence of FMRP, as in FXS, there is a loss of translation suppression and consequent increase in FMRP target mRNA levels, as well as of these mRNAs mGluR-induced [149].

Bear et al. proposed the "mGluR theory" of fragile X, according to which the functional consequences of mGluR-dependent protein synthesis explain the cognitive, behavioral, and physical characteristics observed in this syndrome [70]. *FMR1* is widely expressed throughout the brain, including most cells with postsynaptic mGluRs. Overactivation of mGluRs could explain fragile X symptoms as varied as anxiety, seizures, loose bowel movements, hyperalgesia, obsessive-compulsive symptoms, poor coordination, tactile hypersensitivity, and disturbed sleep patterns [70]. The mGluR theory emerged by the antagonist and non-competitive effects of 6-methyl-2-(phenylethynyl) pyridine (MPEP) on the mGluR5 receptor of Drosophila KO mutants, rescuing short-term memory, abnormal courtship behavior, and mushroom body defects [150, 151].

Extracellular antagonists of mGluRs, particularly mGluR5, have acquired noteworthy interest because they knock down 50% of mGluR5 activity in Fmr1 KO mice. Likewise, blockade of mGluR5 receptors with MPEP in animal models can correct the fragile X cognitive and behavioral phenotype, including propensity toward seizures, increased motor activity, memory impairment, repetitive behavior, sensory-motor processing impairment, and accelerated prepubescent growth [14, 93, 150, 152–154]. Antagonists of mGluR5 have been identified as better therapeutic targets than mGluR1 antagonists since mGluR1 is widely expressed in the cerebellum and, its blockade is associated with motor impairment [14, 149]. However, MPEP is also not specific and leads to significant side effects; therefore, it has not been studied in humans [155].

Table 2. Phase II and III clinical trials in Fragile X syndrome patients

Compound	Mechanism of action	Clinical findings
Fenobam	mGluR5 antagonist	Open-labed, single dose trial in 12 adults: 6/12 (50%) with > 20% improvement in PPI; 9/12 (75%) with observed "calmed" behavior; no effect on attention and response inhibition
AFQ056	mGluR5 antagonist	Randomized, double-blind crossover study in 30 male adults: No improvements on ABC-C subscales in subjects with partial *FMR1* methylation; signification improvement in ABC-C sum score and stereotype; hyperactivity and inappropriate speech subscales in those with full methylation; fatigue and headache common Phase II trials in adults and adolescents and Phase I trials in children underway
Acamprosate	Probable mGluR5 antagonist, $GABA_AR$ agonist and weak NMDA antagonist	Open-label study in 3 adults males: subjective improvement in expressive language skills; no improvement in nonverbal communication Phase III trial in children underway
RO4917523	mGluR5 antagonist	Phase II trial in children underway
STX107	mGluR5 antagonist	Phase II trials in adult males in development
Riluzole	Exact mechanisms unknown, believed to block pre-synaptic glutamate release, enhance glutamate reuptake, block voltage-dependent sodium channels	Open-label study in 6 adult males: 1/6 (16%) with reduction in repetitive behavior and irritability; decreased ERK activation in all patients; 5/6 (83%) with asymptomatic increased in LFTs
Memantine	NMDA antagonist	6 young adults treated with memantine: 4/6 (67%) with improvement on CGI-I; no specific improvement in specific rating scales; 2/6 (33.3%) with treatment-emergent irritability
Minocycline	MMP-9 inhibitor	Open label study in 20 young adults: significant improvement in ABC-C irritability subscale scores; CGI-I and VAS; GI side effects common Phase II trial in children recently completed; results not yet available

Compound	Mechanism of action	Clinical findings
Lithium	GSK3 inhibitor; increases BDNF production	Open label study in 15 children and adults: no improvement in ABC-C irritability subscale scores; mild to moderate improvement in ABC hyperactivity and inappropriate speech subscale scores, CGI-I, VAS and VASB measures; 11/15 (73%) with polyuria/polydipsia; 4/15 (27%) with elevated TSH
Arbaclofen	GABA$_B$R agonist	Phase II randomized, placebo-controlled trial in 63 children and adults: trend toward significance in ABC-C irritability subscale scores and CGI-I scores; 15 severely affected children with significant improvement in CGI-I and ABC social withdrawal subscale scores Phase III trials in children and adults underway
CX516	Positive modulation of AMPA receptors	Randomized, placebo-controlled trials in 49 adults: no improvement on cognitive and behavioral measures
OT	Neuropeptide involved in pro-social behavior	Randomized, placebo-controlled trials in 10 young adult males: increased eye contact during social challenge task at lowest dose; decreased cortisol levels at highest dose
Donepezil	Acetylcholinesterase antagonist	Open label trial in 9 adults: improvement in measures of working memory, cognitive flexibility, hyperactivity, irritability, inattention Randomized controlled trial in young adults underway

ABC-C: Aberrant Behavior Checklist-Community Edition; AMPA: α-amino-3 hidroxy-5 methyl-4-isoxazolepropionic acid; BDNF: Brain derived neurotrophic factor; CGI-I: Clinical Global Impressions Improvement; FXS: Fragile X syndrome; GSK3: Glycogen syntase kinase-3; LFT: Liver function test; mGluR: Metabotrophic glutamate receptor; MMP-9: Matrix metalloproteinase 9; NMDA: N-methyl-D- aspartate; OT: Oxytocin; PPI: Prepulse inhibition; TSH: Thyroid stimulating hormone; VABS: Vineland Adaptative Behavior Scales; VAS: Visual analog scale. Table taken and modified [63].

Validation of the mGluR theory suggests that medications targeting mGluR5 as well as components of the associated signaling cascades could be therapeutic in individuals with FXS [156]. Downstream molecules regulated by the mGluR pathway, including individual proteins, GABARs, AMPARs, and NMDARs, could also be targets for pharmacological intervention. While no medications specifically modulating the mGluR pathway have approval from the Food and Drug Administration (FDA) for treatment in FXS patients, a number of phase II and III trials have been completed or are underway, as will be described in Table 2.

CONCLUSION

Recently, a variety of preclinical studies in animal models have recognized several candidates for treatment of FXS. Such drugs include mGluR antagonists, GABA agonists, minocycline and its derivatives, and targets of the endocannabinoid pathway. Metformin, a well-known and mature antidiabetic drug, has also recently shown beneficial effects in preclinical studies in patients with FXS.

REFERENCES

[1] Martin JP, Bell J. A pedigree of mental defect showing sex-linkage. *J Neurol Psychiatry* 1943; 6: 154–7.

[2] Lubs, H. A., Jr. A marker X chromosome. *Am. J. Hum. Genet.* 1969; 21: 231-244.

[3] Hecht F, Glover TW. Antibiotics containing trimethoprim and the fragile X chromosome. Vol. 308, *The New England journal of medicine*. United States; 1983. p. 285–6.

[4] Steinbach P. Mental impairment in Martin-Bell syndrome is probably determined by interaction of several genes: simple explanation of phenotypic differences between unaffected and affected males with the same X chromosome. *Hum Genet* 1986; 72: 248–52.

[5] Israel MH. Autosomal suppressor gene for fragile-X: an hypothesis. *Am J Med Genet* 1987; 26: 19–31.

[6] Verheij C, Bakker CE, de Graaff E, Keulemans J, Willemsen R, Verkerk AJ, et al. Characterization and localization of the FMR-1 gene product associated with fragile X syndrome. *Nature* 1993; 363: 722–4.

[7] Khandjian EW, Corbin F, Woerly S, Rousseau F. The fragile X mental retardation protein is associated with ribosomes. *Nat Genet* 1996; 12: 91–3.

[8] Oberlé I, Rousseau F, Heitz D, Kretz C, Devys D, Hanauer A, et al. Instability of a 550-base pair DNA segment and abnormal methylation in fragile X syndrome. *Science* 1991; 252: 1097–102.

[9] Yu S, Pritchard M, Kremer E, Lynch M, Nancarrow J, Baker E, et al. Fragile X genotype characterized by an unstable region of DNA. *Science* 1991; 252: 1179–81.

[10] Antar LN, Afroz R, Dictenberg JB, Carroll RC, Bassell GJ. Metabotropic glutamate receptor activation regulates fragile x mental retardation protein and FMR1 mRNA localization differentially in dendrites and at synapses. *J Neurosci* 2004; 24: 2648–55.

[11] Brown V, Jin P, Ceman S, Darnell JC, O'Donnell WT, Tenenbaum SA, et al. Microarray identification of FMRP-associated brain mRNAs and altered mRNA translational profiles in fragile X syndrome. *Cell* 2001; 107: 477–87.

[12] Huber KM, Gallagher SM, Warren ST, Bear MF. Altered synaptic plasticity in a mouse model of fragile X mental retardation. *Proc Natl Acad Sci U S A* 2002; 99: 7746–50.

[13] Gross C, Nakamoto M, Yao X, Chan C-B, Yim SY, Ye K, et al. Excess phosphoinositide 3-kinase subunit synthesis and activity as a novel therapeutic target in fragile X syndrome. *J Neurosci* 2010; 30: 10624–38.

[14] Thomas AM, Bui N, Perkins JR, Yuva-Paylor LA, Paylor R. Group I metabotropic glutamate receptor antagonists alter select behaviors in a mouse model for fragile X syndrome. *Psychopharmacology (Berl)* 2012; 219: 47–58.

[15] Bagni C, Tassone F, Neri G, Hagerman R. Fragile X syndrome: causes, diagnosis, mechanisms, and therapeutics. *J Clin Invest* 2012; 122: 4314–22.

[16] Mila M, Alvarez-Mora MI, Madrigal I, Rodriguez-Revenga L. Fragile X syndrome: An overview and update of the FMR1 gene. *Clin Genet* 2018; 93: 197–205.

[17] Stone WL, Basit H, Los E. Fragile X Syndrome. In *Treasure Island* (FL); 2021.

[18] Liu-Yesucevitz L, Bassell GJ, Gitler AD, Hart AC, Klann E, Richter JD, et al. Local RNA translation at the synapse and in disease. *J Neurosci* 2011; 31: 16086–93.

[19] Rosales-Reynoso MA, Mendoza-Carrera F, Troyo-Sanromán R, Medina C, Barros-Núñez P. Genetic diversity at the FMR1 locus in Mexican population. *Arch Med Res* 2005; 36: 412–7.

[20] Yang W, Fan C, Chen L, Cui Z, Bai Y, Lan F. Pathological Effects of the FMR1 CGG-Repeat Polymorphism (5-55 Repeat Numbers): Systematic Review and Meta-Analysis. *Tohoku J Exp Med* 2016; 239: 57–66.

[21] Nolin SL, Sah S, Glicksman A, Sherman SL, Allen E, Berry-Kravis E, et al. Fragile X AGG analysis provides new risk predictions for 45-69 repeat alleles. *Am J Med Genet A* 2013; 161A: 771–8.

[22] Seltzer MM, Baker MW, Hong J, Maenner M, Greenberg J, Mandel D. Prevalence of CGG expansions of the FMR1 gene in a US population-based sample. *Am J Med Genet Part B, Neuropsychiatr Genet Off Publ Int Soc Psychiatr Genet* 2012; 159B: 589–97.

[23] Turner G, Daniel A, Frost M. X-linked mental retardation, macroorchidism, and the Xq27 fragile site. *J Pediatr* 1980; 96: 837–41.

[24] Hagerman RJ, Van Housen K, Smith AC, McGavran L. Consideration of connective tissue dysfunction in the fragile X syndrome. *Am J Med Genet* 1984; 17: 111–21.

[25] Opitz JM, Sutherland GR. Conference report: International Workshop on the fragile X and X-linked mental retardation. *Am J Med Genet* 1984; 17: 5–94.

[26] Loehr JP, Synhorst DP, Wolfe RR, Hagerman RJ. Aortic root dilatation and mitral valve prolapse in the fragile X syndrome. *Am J Med Genet* 1986; 23: 189–94.

[27] Lozano R, Azarang A, Wilaisakditipakorn T, Hagerman RJ. Fragile X syndrome: A review of clinical management. *Intractable rare Dis Res* 2016; 5: 145–57.

[28] Napoli E, Flores A, Mansuri Y, Hagerman RJ, Giulivi C. Sulforaphane improves mitochondrial metabolism in fibroblasts

from patients with fragile X-associated tremor and ataxia syndrome. *Neurobiol Dis* 2021; 157: 105427.

[29] Kong HE, Zhao J, Xu S, Jin P, Jin Y. Fragile X-Associated Tremor/Ataxia Syndrome: From Molecular Pathogenesis to Development of Therapeutics. *Front Cell Neurosci* 2017; 11: 128.

[30] Cao Y, Peng Y, Kong HE, Allen EG, Jin P. Metabolic Alterations in FMR1 Premutation Carriers. *Front Mol Biosci* 2020; 7: 571092.

[31] Malecki C, Hambly BD, Jeremy RW, Robertson EN. The RNA-binding fragile-X mental retardation protein and its role beyond the brain. *Biophys Rev* 2020; 12: 903–16.

[32] Man L, Lekovich J, Rosenwaks Z, Gerhardt J. Fragile X-Associated Diminished Ovarian Reserve and Primary Ovarian Insufficiency from Molecular Mechanisms to Clinical Manifestations. *Front Mol Neurosci* 2017; 10: 290.

[33] Hagerman RJ, Berry-Kravis E, Hazlett HC, Bailey DBJ, Moine H, Kooy RF, et al. Fragile X syndrome. *Nat Rev Dis Prim* 2017; 3: 17065.

[34] Hagerman RJ, Hagerman P. Fragile X-associated tremor/ataxia syndrome - features, mechanisms and management. *Nat Rev Neurol* 2016; 12: 403–12.

[35] Nolin SL, Glicksman A, Ersalesi N, Dobkin C, Brown WT, Cao R, et al. Fragile X full mutation expansions are inhibited by one or more AGG interruptions in premutation carriers. *Genet Med* 2015; 17: 358–64.

[36] Verkerk AJ, Pieretti M, Sutcliffe JS, Fu YH, Kuhl DP, Pizzuti A, et al. Identification of a gene (FMR-1) containing a CGG repeat coincident with a breakpoint cluster region exhibiting length variation in fragile X syndrome. *Cell* 1991; 65: 905–14.

[37] Eichler EE, Richards S, Gibbs RA, Nelson DL. Fine structure of the human FMR1 gene. *Hum Mol Genet* 1993; 2: 1147–53.

[38] Brackett DM, Qing F, Amieux PS, Sellers DL, Horner PJ, Morris DR. FMR1 transcript isoforms: association with polyribosomes; regional and developmental expression in mouse brain. *PLoS One* 2013; 8: e58296.

[39] Pretto DI, Eid JS, Yrigollen CM, Tang H-T, Loomis EW, Raske C, et al. Differential increases of specific FMR1 mRNA isoforms in premutation carriers. *J Med Genet* 2015; 52: 42–52.

[40] Adinolfi S, Bagni C, Musco G, Gibson T, Mazzarella L, Pastore A. Dissecting FMR1, the protein responsible for fragile X syndrome, in its structural and functional domains. *RNA* 1999; 5: 1248–58.

[41] Adinolfi S, Ramos A, Martin SR, Dal Piaz F, Pucci P, Bardoni B, et al. The N-terminus of the fragile X mental retardation protein contains a novel domain involved in dimerization and RNA binding. *Biochemistry* 2003; 42: 10437–44.

[42] Darnell JC, Van Driesche SJ, Zhang C, Hung KYS, Mele A, Fraser CE, et al. FMRP stalls ribosomal translocation on mRNAs linked to synaptic function and autism. *Cell* 2011; 146: 247–61.

[43] Sidorov MS, Auerbach BD, Bear MF. Fragile X mental retardation protein and synaptic plasticity. *Mol Brain* 2013; 6: 15.

[44] Devys D, Lutz Y, Rouyer N, Bellocq JP, Mandel JL. The FMR-1 protein is cytoplasmic, most abundant in neurons and appears normal in carriers of a fragile X premutation. *Nat Genet* 1993; 4: 335–40.

[45] Hinds HL, Ashley CT, Sutcliffe JS, Nelson DL, Warren ST, Housman DE, et al. Tissue specific expression of FMR-1 provides evidence for a functional role in fragile X syndrome. *Nat Genet* 1993; 3: 36–43.

[46] Santoro MR, Bray SM, Warren ST. Molecular mechanisms of fragile X syndrome: a twenty-year perspective. *Annu Rev Pathol* 2012; 7: 219–45.

[47] Ashley CTJ, Wilkinson KD, Reines D, Warren ST. FMR1 protein: conserved RNP family domains and selective RNA binding. *Science* 1993; 262: 563–6.

[48] Bechara EG, Didiot MC, Melko M, Davidovic L, Bensaid M, Martin P, et al. A novel function for fragile X mental retardation protein in translational activation. *PLoS Biol* 2009; 7: e16.

[49] Stefani G, Fraser CE, Darnell JC, Darnell RB. Fragile X mental retardation protein is associated with translating polyribosomes in neuronal cells. *J Neurosci* 2004; 24: 7272–6.

[50] Darnell JC, Mostovetsky O, Darnell RB. FMRP RNA targets: identification and validation. *Genes Brain Behav* 2005; 4: 341–9.

[51] Laggerbauer B, Ostareck D, Keidel EM, Ostareck-Lederer A, Fischer U. Evidence that fragile X mental retardation protein is a negative regulator of translation. *Hum Mol Genet* 2001; 10: 329–38.

[52] Siomi H, Choi M, Siomi MC, Nussbaum RL, Dreyfuss G. Essential role for KH domains in RNA binding: impaired RNA binding by a mutation in the KH domain of FMR1 that causes fragile X syndrome. *Cell* 1994; 77: 33–9.

[53] Tian H, Cao Y-X, Zhang X-S, Liao W-P, Yi Y-H, Lian J, et al. The targeting and functions of miRNA-383 are mediated by FMRP during spermatogenesis. *Cell Death Dis* 2013; 4: e617.

[54] Lacoux C, Di Marino D, Boyl PP, Zalfa F, Yan B, Ciotti MT, et al. BC1-FMRP interaction is modulated by 2'-O-methylation: RNA-binding activity of the tudor domain and translational regulation at synapses. *Nucleic Acids Res* 2012; 40: 4086–96.

[55] Wang T, Bray SM, Warren ST. New perspectives on the biology of fragile X syndrome. *Curr Opin Genet Dev* 2012; 22: 256–63.

[56] Banerjee A, Ifrim MF, Valdez AN, Raj N, Bassell GJ. Aberrant RNA translation in fragile X syndrome: From FMRP mechanisms to emerging therapeutic strategies. *Brain Res* 2018; 1693: 24–36.

[57] Ascano MJ, Mukherjee N, Bandaru P, Miller JB, Nusbaum JD, Corcoran DL, et al. FMRP targets distinct mRNA sequence elements to regulate protein expression. *Nature* 2012; 492: 382–6.

[58] Darnell JC, Richter JD. Cytoplasmic RNA-binding proteins and the control of complex brain function. *Cold Spring Harb Perspect Biol* 2012; 4: a012344.

[59] Oostra BA, Willemsen R. FMR1: a gene with three faces. *Biochim Biophys Acta* 2009; 1790: 467–77.

[60] Gantois I, Vandesompele J, Speleman F, Reyniers E, D'Hooge R, Severijnen L-A, et al. Expression profiling suggests

underexpression of the GABA(A) receptor subunit delta in the fragile X knockout mouse model. *Neurobiol Dis* 2006; 21: 346–57.

[61] De Rubeis S, Bagni C. Fragile X mental retardation protein control of neuronal mRNA metabolism: Insights into mRNA stability. *Mol Cell Neurosci* 2010; 43: 43–50.

[62] Zhang M, Wang Q, Huang Y. Fragile X mental retardation protein FMRP and the RNA export factor NXF2 associate with and destabilize Nxf1 mRNA in neuronal cells. *Proc Natl Acad Sci U S A* 2007; 104: 10057–62.

[63] Barros-Núñez Patricio, Rosales-Reynoso Mónica-Alejandra, and Juárez-Vázquez CI. Therapeutic Approaches to Fragile X Syndrome. In: Urbano. K V., editor. *Advances in Genetics Research* Nova Science Publishers; 2014. p. 153–82.

[64] Kanai Y, Dohmae N, Hirokawa N. Kinesin transports RNA: isolation and characterization of an RNA-transporting granule. *Neuron* 2004; 43: 513–25.

[65] Ferrari F, Mercaldo V, Piccoli G, Sala C, Cannata S, Achsel T, et al. The fragile X mental retardation protein-RNP granules show an mGluR-dependent localization in the post-synaptic spines. *Mol Cell Neurosci* 2007; 34: 343–54.

[66] Charalambous DC, Pasciuto E, Mercaldo V, Pilo Boyl P, Munck S, Bagni C, et al. KIF1Bβ transports dendritically localized mRNPs in neurons and is recruited to synapses in an activity-dependent manner. *Cell Mol Life Sci* 2013; 70: 335–56.

[67] Muddashetty RS, Kelić S, Gross C, Xu M, Bassell GJ. Dysregulated metabotropic glutamate receptor-dependent translation of AMPA receptor and postsynaptic density-95 mRNAs at synapses in a mouse model of fragile X syndrome. *J Neurosci* 2007; 27: 5338–48.

[68] De Rubeis S, Pasciuto E, Li KW, Fernández E, Di Marino D, Buzzi A, et al. CYFIP1 coordinates mRNA translation and cytoskeleton remodeling to ensure proper dendritic spine formation. *Neuron* 2013; 79: 1169–82.

[69] Fernández E, Rajan N, Bagni C. The FMRP regulon: from targets to disease convergence. *Front Neurosci* 2013; 7: 191.

[70] Bear MF, Huber KM, Warren ST. The mGluR theory of fragile X mental retardation. *Trends Neurosci* 2004; 27: 370–7.

[71] Kao DI, Aldridge GM, Weiler IJ, Greenough WT. Altered mRNA transport, docking, and protein translation in neurons lacking fragile X mental retardation protein. *Proc Natl Acad Sci U S A* 2010; 107: 15601–6.

[72] Hou L, Antion MD, Hu D, Spencer CM, Paylor R, Klann E. Dynamic translational and proteasomal regulation of fragile X mental retardation protein controls mGluR-dependent long-term depression. *Neuron* 2006; 51: 441–54.

[73] Ceman S, O'Donnell WT, Reed M, Patton S, Pohl J, Warren ST. Phosphorylation influences the translation state of FMRP-associated polyribosomes. *Hum Mol Genet* 2003; 12: 3295–305.

[74] Narayanan U, Nalavadi V, Nakamoto M, Pallas DC, Ceman S, Bassell GJ, et al. FMRP phosphorylation reveals an immediate-early signaling pathway triggered by group I mGluR and mediated by PP2A. *J Neurosci* 2007; 27: 14349–57.

[75] Papoulas O, Monzo KF, Cantin GT, Ruse C, Yates JR 3rd, Ryu YH, et al. dFMRP and Caprin, translational regulators of synaptic plasticity, control the cell cycle at the Drosophila mid-blastula transition. *Development* 2010; 137: 4201–9.

[76] Napoli I, Mercaldo V, Boyl PP, Eleuteri B, Zalfa F, De Rubeis S, et al. The fragile X syndrome protein represses activity-dependent translation through CYFIP1, a new 4E-BP. *Cell* 2008; 134: 1042–54.

[77] Edens BM, Vissers C, Su J, Arumugam S, Xu Z, Shi H, et al. FMRP Modulates Neural Differentiation through m(6)A-Dependent mRNA Nuclear Export. *Cell Rep* 2019; 28: 845-854.e5.

[78] Alpatov R, Lesch BJ, Nakamoto-Kinoshita M, Blanco A, Chen S, Stützer A, et al. A chromatin-dependent role of the fragile X mental retardation protein FMRP in the DNA damage response. *Cell* 2014; 157: 869–81.

[79] Sittler A, Devys D, Weber C, Mandel JL. Alternative splicing of exon 14 determines nuclear or cytoplasmic localisation of fmr1 protein isoforms. *Hum Mol Genet* 1996; 5: 95–102.

[80] Darnell JC, Klann E. The translation of translational control by FMRP: therapeutic targets for FXS. *Nat Neurosci* 2013; 16: 1530-6.

[81] Richter JD, Bassell GJ, Klann E. Dysregulation and restoration of translational homeostasis in fragile X syndrome. *Nat Rev Neurosci* 2015; 16: 595–605.

[82] Brown MR, Kronengold J, Gazula V-R, Chen Y, Strumbos JG, Sigworth FJ, et al. Fragile X mental retardation protein controls gating of the sodium-activated potassium channel Slack. *Nat Neurosci* 2010; 13: 819–21.

[83] Deng PY, Rotman Z, Blundon JA, Cho Y, Cui J, Cavalli V, et al. FMRP regulates neurotransmitter release and synaptic information transmission by modulating action potential duration via BK channels. *Neuron* 2013; 77: 696–711.

[84] Shamay-Ramot A, Khermesh K, Porath HT, Barak M, Pinto Y, Wachtel C, et al. Fmrp Interacts with Adar and Regulates RNA Editing, Synaptic Density and Locomotor Activity in Zebrafish. *PLoS Genet* 2015; 11: e1005702.

[85] Guo W, Allan AM, Zong R, Zhang L, Johnson EB, Schaller EG, et al. Ablation of Fmrp in adult neural stem cells disrupts hippocampus-dependent learning. *Nat Med* 2011; 17: 559–65.

[86] Akins MR, Leblanc HF, Stackpole EE, Chyung E, Fallon JR. Systematic mapping of fragile X granules in the mouse brain reveals a potential role for presynaptic FMRP in sensorimotor functions. *J Comp Neurol* 2012; 520: 3687–706.

[87] Kaufmann WE, Kidd SA, Andrews HF, Budimirovic DB, Esler A, Haas-Givler B, et al. Autism Spectrum Disorder in Fragile X Syndrome: Cooccurring Conditions and Current Treatment. *Pediatrics* 2017; 139: S194–206.

[88] Braat S, Kooy RF. Fragile X syndrome neurobiology translates into rational therapy. *Drug Discov Today* 2014; 19: 510–9.

[89] Pop AS, Gomez-Mancilla B, Neri G, Willemsen R, Gasparini F. Fragile X syndrome: a preclinical review on metabotropic glutamate receptor 5 (mGluR5) antagonists and drug development. *Psychopharmacology* (Berl) 2014; 231: 1217–26.

[90] Pfeiffer BE, Huber KM. Current advances in local protein synthesis and synaptic plasticity. *J Neurosci* 2006; 26: 7147–50.

[91] Sutton MA, Schuman EM. Dendritic protein synthesis, synaptic plasticity, and memory. *Cell* 2006; 127: 49–58.

[92] Qin M, Kang J, Burlin T V, Jiang C, Smith CB. Postadolescent changes in regional cerebral protein synthesis: an in vivo study in the FMR1 null mouse. *J Neurosci* 2005; 25: 5087–95.

[93] Dölen G, Osterweil E, Rao BSS, Smith GB, Auerbach BD, Chattarji S, et al. Correction of fragile X syndrome in mice. *Neuron* 2007; 56: 955–62.

[94] Braat S, Kooy RF. Insights into GABAAergic system deficits in fragile X syndrome lead to clinical trials. *Neuropharmacology* 2015; 88: 48–54.

[95] Gross C, Chang C-W, Kelly SM, Bhattacharya A, McBride SMJ, Danielson SW, et al. Increased expression of the PI3K enhancer PIKE mediates deficits in synaptic plasticity and behavior in fragile X syndrome. *Cell Rep* 2015; 11: 727–36.

[96] Gkogkas CG, Khoutorsky A, Cao R, Jafarnejad SM, Prager-Khoutorsky M, Giannakas N, et al. Pharmacogenetic inhibition of eIF4E-dependent Mmp9 mRNA translation reverses fragile X syndrome-like phenotypes. *Cell Rep* 2014; 9: 1742–55.

[97] Guo W, Murthy AC, Zhang L, Johnson EB, Schaller EG, Allan AM, et al. Inhibition of GSK3beta improves hippocampus-dependent learning and rescues neurogenesis in a mouse model of fragile X syndrome. *Hum Mol Genet* 2012; 21: 681–91.

[98] Westmark CJ, Westmark PR, O'Riordan KJ, Ray BC, Hervey CM, Salamat MS, et al. Reversal of fragile X phenotypes by manipulation of AβPP/Aβ levels in Fmr1KO mice. *PLoS One* 2011; 6: e26549.

[99] Tabet R, Vitale N, Moine H. Fragile X syndrome: Are signaling lipids the missing culprits? *Biochimie* 2016; 130: 188–94.

[100] Pasciuto E, Ahmed T, Wahle T, Gardoni F, D'Andrea L, Pacini L, et al. Dysregulated ADAM10-Mediated Processing of APP during a Critical Time Window Leads to Synaptic Deficits in Fragile X Syndrome. *Neuron* 2015; 87: 382–98.

[101] Michaluk P, Wawrzyniak M, Alot P, Szczot M, Wyrembek P, Mercik K, et al. Influence of matrix metalloproteinase MMP-9 on dendritic spine morphology. *J Cell Sci* 2011; 124: 3369–80.

[102] Dziembowska M, Pretto DI, Janusz A, Kaczmarek L, Leigh MJ, Gabriel N, et al. High MMP-9 activity levels in fragile X syndrome are lowered by minocycline. *Am J Med Genet A* 2013; 161A: 1897–903.

[103] Bilousova T V, Dansie L, Ngo M, Aye J, Charles JR, Ethell DW, et al. Minocycline promotes dendritic spine maturation and improves behavioural performance in the fragile X mouse model. *J Med Genet* 2009; 46: 94–102.

[104] Gantois I, Khoutorsky A, Popic J, Aguilar-Valles A, Freemantle E, Cao R, et al. Metformin ameliorates core deficits in a mouse model of fragile X syndrome. *Nat Med* 2017; 23: 674–7.

[105] Imai S, Kai M, Yasuda S, Kanoh H, Sakane F. Identification and characterization of a novel human type II diacylglycerol kinase, DGK kappa. *J Biol Chem* 2005; 280: 39870–81.

[106] Sakane F, Imai S, Kai M, Yasuda S, Kanoh H. Diacylglycerol kinases as emerging potential drug targets for a variety of diseases. *Curr Drug Targets* 2008; 9: 626–40.

[107] Kim K, Yang J, Kim E. Diacylglycerol kinases in the regulation of dendritic spines. *J Neurochem* 2010; 112: 577–87.

[108] Pacher P, Bátkai S, Kunos G. The endocannabinoid system as an emerging target of pharmacotherapy. *Pharmacol Rev* 2006; 58: 389–462.

[109] Mouslech Z, Valla V. Endocannabinoid system: An overview of its potential in current medical practice. *Neuro Endocrinol Lett* 2009; 30: 153–79.

[110] Zhang L, Alger BE. Enhanced endocannabinoid signaling elevates neuronal excitability in fragile X syndrome. *J Neurosci* 2010; 30: 5724–9.

[111] Maccarrone M, Gasperi V, Catani MV, Diep TA, Dainese E, Hansen HS, et al. The endocannabinoid system and its relevance for nutrition. *Annu Rev Nutr* 2010; 30: 423–40.

[112] Busquets-Garcia A, Gomis-González M, Guegan T, Agustín-Pavón C, Pastor A, Mato S, et al. Targeting the endocannabinoid system in the treatment of fragile X syndrome. *Nat Med* 2013; 19: 603–7.

[113] Jung K-M, Clapper JR, Fu J, D'Agostino G, Guijarro A, Thongkham D, et al. 2-arachidonoylglycerol signaling in forebrain regulates systemic energy metabolism. *Cell Metab* 2012; 15: 299–310.

[114] Contractor A, Klyachko VA, Portera-Cailliau C. Altered Neuronal and Circuit Excitability in Fragile X Syndrome. *Neuron* 2015; 87: 699–715.

[115] Olmos-Serrano JL, Paluszkiewicz SM, Martin BS, Kaufmann WE, Corbin JG, Huntsman MM. Defective GABAergic neurotransmission and pharmacological rescue of neuronal hyperexcitability in the amygdala in a mouse model of fragile X syndrome. *J Neurosci* 2010; 30: 9929–38.

[116] Vislay RL, Martin BS, Olmos-Serrano JL, Kratovac S, Nelson DL, Corbin JG, et al. Homeostatic responses fail to correct defective amygdala inhibitory circuit maturation in fragile X syndrome. *J Neurosci* 2013; 33: 7548–58.

[117] Sabanov V, Braat S, D'Andrea L, Willemsen R, Zeidler S, Rooms L, et al. Impaired GABAergic inhibition in the hippocampus of Fmr1 knockout mice. *Neuropharmacology* 2017; 116: 71–81.

[118] He Q, Nomura T, Xu J, Contractor A. The developmental switch in GABA polarity is delayed in fragile X mice. *J Neurosci* 2014; 34: 446–50.

[119] Lozano R, Hare EB, Hagerman RJ. Modulation of the GABAergic pathway for the treatment of fragile X syndrome. *Neuropsychiatr Dis Treat* 2014; 10: 1769–79.

[120] Chang S, Bray SM, Li Z, Zarnescu DC, He C, Jin P, et al. Identification of small molecules rescuing fragile X syndrome phenotypes in *Drosophila*. *Nat Chem Biol* 2008; 4: 256–63.

[121] Reddy DS, Estes WA. Clinical Potential of Neurosteroids for CNS Disorders. *Trends Pharmacol Sci* 2016; 37: 543–61.

[122] Braat S, Kooy RF. The GABAA Receptor as a Therapeutic Target for Neurodevelopmental Disorders. *Neuron* 2015; 86: 1119–30.

[123] Tyzio R, Nardou R, Ferrari DC, Tsintsadze T, Shahrokhi A, Eftekhari S, et al. Oxytocin-mediated GABA inhibition during delivery attenuates autism pathogenesis in rodent offspring. *Science* 2014; 343: 675–9.

[124] Blavier L, Delaissé JM. Matrix metalloproteinases are obligatory for the migration of preosteoclasts to the developing marrow cavity of primitive long bones. *J Cell Sci* 1995; 108 (Pt 1: 3649–59.

[125] Janusz A, Milek J, Perycz M, Pacini L, Bagni C, Kaczmarek L, et al. The Fragile X mental retardation protein regulates matrix metalloproteinase 9 mRNA at synapses. *J Neurosci* 2013; 33: 18234–41.

[126] Luca R, Averna M, Zalfa F, Vecchi M, Bianchi F, La Fata G, et al. The fragile X protein binds mRNAs involved in cancer progression and modulates metastasis formation. *EMBO Mol Med* 2013; 5: 1523–36.

[127] Sidhu TS, French SL, Hamilton JR. Differential signaling by protease-activated receptors: implications for therapeutic targeting. *Int J Mol Sci* 2014; 15: 6169–83.

[128] Leigh MJS, Nguyen D V, Mu Y, Winarni TI, Schneider A, Chechi T, et al. A randomized double-blind, placebo-controlled trial of minocycline in children and adolescents with fragile x syndrome. *J Dev Behav Pediatr* 2013; 34: 147–55.

[129] Siller SS, Broadie K. Matrix metalloproteinases and minocycline: therapeutic avenues for fragile X syndrome. *Neural Plast* 2012; 2012: 124548.

[130] Zalfa F, Panasiti V, Carotti S, Zingariello M, Perrone G, Sancillo L, et al. The fragile X mental retardation protein regulates tumor

invasiveness-related pathways in melanoma cells. *Cell Death Dis* 2017; 8: e3169.

[131] Li L, Zeng Q, Bhutkar A, Galván JA, Karamitopoulou E, Noordermeer D, et al. GKAP Acts as a Genetic Modulator of NMDAR Signaling to Govern Invasive Tumor Growth. *Cancer Cell* 2018; 33: 736-751.e5.

[132] Li Y, Tang Y, Ye L, Liu B, Liu K, Chen J, et al. Establishment of a hepatocellular carcinoma cell line with unique metastatic characteristics through in vivo selection and screening for metastasis-related genes through cDNA microarray. *J Cancer Res Clin Oncol* 2003; 129: 43–51.

[133] Liu Y, Zhu X, Zhu J, Liao S, Tang Q, Liu K, et al. Identification of differential expression of genes in hepatocellular carcinoma by suppression subtractive hybridization combined cDNA microarray. *Oncol Rep* 2007; 18: 943–51.

[134] Kalkunte R, Macarthur D, Morton R. Glioblastoma in a boy with fragile X: an unusual case of neuroprotection. *Arch Dis Child* 2007; 92: 795–6.

[135] Schultz-Pedersen S, Hasle H, Olsen JH, Friedrich U. Evidence of decreased risk of cancer in individuals with fragile X. *Am J Med Genet* 2001; 103: 226–30.

[136] Rosales Reynoso MA, Ochoa Hernandez AB, Aguilar Lemarroy A, Jave Suarez LF, Troyo Sanroman R, Barros Nunez P. Gene expression profiling identifies WNT7A as a possible candidate gene for decreased cancer risk in fragile X syndrome patients. *Arch Med Res* 2010; 41: 110-118.e2.

[137] Lucá R, Averna M, Zalfa F, Vecchi M, Bianchi F, La Fata G, et al. The fragile X protein binds mRNAs involved in cancer progression and modulates metastasis formation. *EMBO Mol Med* 2013; 5: 1523–36.

[138] Zhu YJ, Zheng B, Luo GJ, Ma XK, Lu XY, Lin XM, et al. Circular RNAs negatively regulate cancer stem cells by physically binding FMRP against CCAR1 complex in hepatocellular carcinoma. *Theranostics* 2019; 9: 3526–40.

[139] Van Dijck A, Barbosa S, Bermudez-Martin P, Khalfallah O, Gilet C, Martinuzzi E, et al. Reduced serum levels of pro-inflammatory chemokines in fragile X syndrome. *BMC Neurol* 2020; 20: 138.

[140] Shen A, Wu M, Liu L, Chen Y, Chen X, Zhuang M, et al. Targeting NUFIP1 Suppresses Growth and Induces Senescence of Colorectal Cancer Cells. *Front Oncol* 2021; 11: 681425.

[141] Di Grazia A, Marafini I, Pedini G, Di Fusco D, Laudisi F, Dinallo V, et al. The Fragile X Mental Retardation Protein Regulates RIPK1 and Colorectal Cancer Resistance to Necroptosis. *Cell Mol Gastroenterol Hepatol* 2021; 11: 639–58.

[142] Bardoni B, Abekhoukh S, Zongaro S, Melko M. Intellectual disabilities, neuronal posttranscriptional RNA metabolism, and RNA-binding proteins: three actors for a complex scenario. *Prog Brain Res* 2012; 197: 29–51.

[143] Didiot MC, Tian Z, Schaeffer C, Subramanian M, Mandel JL, Moine H. The G-quartet containing FMRP binding site in FMR1 mRNA is a potent exonic splicing enhancer. *Nucleic Acids Res* 2008; 36: 4902–12.

[144] Maurin T, Zongaro S, Bardoni B. Fragile X Syndrome: from molecular pathology to therapy. *Neurosci Biobehav Rev* 2014; 46 Pt 2: 242–55.

[145] Majumder M, Johnson RH, Palanisamy V. Fragile X-related protein family: a double-edged sword in neurodevelopmental disorders and cancer. *Crit Rev Biochem Mol Biol* 2020; 55: 409–24.

[146] Cammas A, Millevoi S. RNA G-quadruplexes: emerging mechanisms in disease. *Nucleic Acids Res* 2017; 45: 1584–95.

[147] Papa L, Manfredi G, Germain D. SOD1, an unexpected novel target for cancer therapy. *Genes Cancer* 2014; 5: 15–21.

[148] Dölen G, Carpenter RL, Ocain TD, Bear MF. Mechanism-based approaches to treating fragile X. *Pharmacol Ther* 2010; 127: 78–93.

[149] Berry-Kravis E, Knox A, Hervey C. Targeted treatments for fragile X syndrome. *J Neurodev Disord* 2011; 3: 193–210.

[150] McBride SMJ, Choi CH, Wang Y, Liebelt D, Braunstein E, Ferreiro D, et al. Pharmacological rescue of synaptic plasticity, courtship

behavior, and mushroom body defects in a *Drosophila* model of fragile X syndrome. *Neuron* 2005; 45: 753-64.

[151] Dölen G, Bear MF. Courting a cure for fragile X. *Neuron* 2005; 45: 642-4.

[152] Westmark CJ, Westmark PR, Malter JS. MPEP reduces seizure severity in Fmr-1 KO mice over expressing human Abeta. *Int J Clin Exp Pathol* 2009; 3: 56-68.

[153] Yan QJ, Rammal M, Tranfaglia M, Bauchwitz RP. Suppression of two major Fragile X Syndrome mouse model phenotypes by the mGluR5 antagonist MPEP. *Neuropharmacology* 2005; 49: 1053-66.

[154] de Vrij FMS, Levenga J, van der Linde HC, Koekkoek SK, De Zeeuw CI, Nelson DL, et al. Rescue of behavioral phenotype and neuronal protrusion morphology in Fmr1 KO mice. *Neurobiol Dis* 2008; 31: 127-32.

[155] Levenga J, Hayashi S, de Vrij FMS, Koekkoek SK, van der Linde HC, Nieuwenhuizen I, et al. AFQ056, a new mGluR5 antagonist for treatment of fragile X syndrome. *Neurobiol Dis* 2011; 42: 311-7.

[156] Bear MF. Therapeutic implications of the mGluR theory of fragile X mental retardation. *Genes Brain Behav* 2005; 4: 393-8.

In: Fragile X Syndrome
Editor: Fabrizio Stasolla

ISBN: 978-1-68507-572-9
© 2022 Nova Science Publishers, Inc.

Chapter 2

FRAGILE X SYNDROME: COMMON NEUROPSYCHIATRIC ASSOCIATIONS

Silvina Tonarelli[1,2,*] *and Zarin Akhter*[1,2]

[1]Psychiatry Department,
Texas Tech University Health Science Center,
El Paso, TX, USA
[2]Paul L Foster School of Medicine, El Paso, TX, USA

ABSTRACT

Background

Fragile X Syndrome (FXS) is a trinucleotic repeat disorder either caused by a lack or deficiency of a protein called *fragile X*. Lack of this protein results in mental retardation and the protein is involved in development and maintenance of neuronal synaptic connections. FXS is an X-linked disorder and it is associated with inherited intellectual disabilities, as well as autism spectrum disorder.

---

[*] Corresponding Author's E-mail: silvina.tonarelli@ttuhsc.edu.

Objectives

This chapter describes the most common neuropsychiatric conditions associated to Fragile X Syndrome.

Method

We performed a critical review of the literature and here we summarized the data on FXS and its impact on neuropsychiatric disorders.

Results

Fragile X Syndrome is commonly associated to intellectual disabilities, autism spectrum disorder, anxiety disorders, and attention deficit-hyperactivity disorder. Additionally, learning disorders, seizures, and language deficit disorders are also observed in individuals with FXS. Other characteristics associated with FXS include: obsessive compulsive disorder, mood swings, impulse control behavior, and stereotypies such as hand flapping or biting. Some individuals have cognitive deficits in the areas of short-term and working memory, visuospatial and mathematic abilities, and executive functions. Lastly, it is rare for patients with FXS to present with catatonia and psychosis.

Conclusion

The clinical presentation of FXS is heterogeneous with variations in severity and symptomology depending on age, gender, and if the mutation is partial or full. Disorders of anxiety and social withdrawal are the core features of the FXS. FXS is frequently associated with learning disabilities, attention-deficit hyperactivity disorder, and epilepsy. In conclusion, optimal diagnosis of FXS includes screening for neuropsychiatric disorders in order to customize treatment to reduce comorbidities.

Keywords: fragile X syndrome, neuropsychiatry, intellectual disability, autism, ADHD

1. INTRODUCTION

Fragile X Syndrome (FXS) is a trinucleotic repeat disorder caused by excessive cytosine-guanine-guanine (CGG) repeats on the fragile X mental retardation 1 (FMR1) gene located on the Xq27.3 site. Individuals can present with either a full mutation (more than 200 CGG repeats on the FMR1 gene) or a premutation (55-200 CGG repeats). A consequence of CGG repeats is a lack or deficiency of a protein called fragile X mental retardation protein (FMRP). The FMRP regulates gene expression of genes involved in the development and maintenance of neuronal synaptic connections [1, 2].

Patients with FXS exhibit physical characteristics which vary depending on the disease severity and whether there is a full mutation or a premutation. The most common phenotypic traits are noted to be an enlargement of the ears and head, short stature, hyperextensible joints, high arched palate, decreased muscle tone, and a post-pubertal macroorchidism [3]. FXS is a neurogenetic disease with cognitive-behavioral manifestations. Early detection of neuropsychiatric conditions is essential in order to optimize the long-term outcomes of those with FXS.

Understanding the pathophysiology and phenotype of FXS can be complex because there are overlapping, dynamic interactions among neuropsychiatric manifestations. Additional challenges in the diagnosis of comorbidities are related to a patient's limitations on language, self-awareness, and cognitive skills necessary for complete assessment of the neuropsychiatric disorders. Further adding to the complexity of the disorder are interactions at the genetic, molecular, cellular, and neurocircuit/physiology levels which impact behavior within this complex disorder [4].

Data from a national survey of children with FXS shows that the most common neuropsychiatric conditions associated with full mutations are intellectual disability (ID), autism spectrum disorder (ASD), anxiety, and attentional deficit-hyperactivity disorder (ADHD). Learning disorders, seizures, and language function disorders are also observed in children with FXS. Obsessive compulsive disorder, mood swings, impulse control behavior, and stereotypies like hand flapping or biting are commonly observed in these patients. Individuals can have cognitive deficits in the areas of short-term and working memory, visuospatial and mathematic abilities, and executive functions [5]. Rarely, patients can present with catatonia and psychosis [6, 7]. Frequently, multiple neuropsychiatric co-morbidities are present together in the same patient [8-10].

In this chapter, we critically review the available evidence of the most common neuropsychiatric associations seen in patients with FXS. The overlap of symptoms and their variable courses during their life spans are some of the challenges in correcting diagnoses of these disorders.

2. INTELLECTUAL DISABILITY AND AUTISM SPECTRUM DISORDERS

The expression of FXS varies between males and females. ID and ASD are more commonly found in males who have full mutation FXS when compared to FXS females. Females on the other hand present predominantly with learning disorders (60%) when compared to FXS males. Additionally, males are reported to have dysfunctions in working memory, visuospatial and mathematic abilities, and executive functions. These deficits are more severe in FXS boys with autistic behaviors [5, 11].

FXS is associated with reductions in cognition. De Vries et al. [12], studied the intelligence quotients (IQ) in 33 adult females with full mutations and compared them to a control group of 28 first degree relatives without full mutations. The author reported that approximately 70% of the FXS female subjects with full mutations had IQ scores of less than 85; whereas in FXS males with full mutations the IQ was reported to be 40 and those males with premutations typically had normal to borderline IQs. More concerningly, even in the subjects with FXS who had normal IQs, emotional deficits could be present [12].

2.1. Anxiety

Anxiety disorders and social withdrawal are considered core features of the FXS phenotype. The most common types of anxiety disorders are generalized anxiety disorder, social phobia, specific phobia, selective mutism, and separation anxiety. Among FXS males, 80% meet the criteria for one anxiety disorder and 60% have several anxiety disorders. Patients with FXS have dysregulated, persistently high fear in response to low levels of threat. However, despite this dysregulation, patients with FXS still like to interact with others [13]. At least 50% of adolescents with FXS have anxiety. Cordeiro, L., et al., [15] studied premutation carrying children and adolescents (ages 5-23 years) and found approximately 70.6% of the subjects met the criteria for at least one anxiety disorder (most frequently generalized anxiety disorder, specific phobia, social phobia, or obsessive compulsive disorder), compared to 22.6% of the control group, and 9.8% of the general population in a comparable age range. The highest rate of anxiety was associated with intellectual disability, male gender, and proband status; however, non-probands also had higher rates anxiety disorders (40.0%) when compared to the general population. The National Fragile X Survey provided information on comorbidities in 1,027 male children (ages 3-11) with FXS and their data suggested that autism and anxiety disorders were the most prevalent in FXS. Additionally, they found individuals with FXS also suffered from symptoms compatible with ADHD (attention problems and hyperactivity/impulsivity), aggression, and self-injurious behavior. In order to begin understanding these underlying conditions associated with the psychopathology of anxiety and ASD in FXS children, Wall et al., [16] examined the trajectory from infancy through preschool in males and females with FXS and found that negative temperamental effects were an early marker for anxiety in young children with FXS.

2.2. Social Anxiety

FXS is commonly associated with higher social anxiety and social communication difficulties compared with other neurodevelopmental disorders. In order to identify social anxiety early in life, Black et al., [19] studied infants with FXS and observed that at 12 months old there appeared to be an elevation in behavioral inhibition, increased attention towards strangers, and physiological dysregulation, such as a blunted respiratory sinus arrhythmia response. The authors concluded these were early markers of social anxiety in this population. Interestingly, FXS patients have preserved social motivation [14, 15], as demonstrated by

Scherr et al., [20] who investigated preschool children with FXS and found that distinct behavioral patterns regarding social anxiety or fear of strangers were observed depending on the degree of severity of ASD. For example, boys with more severe ASD demonstrated more avoidance gaze and less eye contact with strangers when compared to those with low functioning autism.

3. SOCIAL COMMUNICATION AND SOCIAL SKILLS

Social skills are critical for academic, social, and psychological success of children. Boys with FXS are at high risk for social skill impairments due in large part to intellectual disabilities and the other comorbidities commonly associated with FXS. McDuffie and colleagues [22] found boys with FXS are less impaired in social smiling and more impaired in complex mannerisms when compared to boys with non-syndromic ASD. McDuffie et al., also studied two different indexes of object play skills in 10 male toddlers with FXS to evaluate the nonverbal communication of children interacting with their mothers in play. The results of this study showed that the object interest index, or number of toys touched, was positively related to standardized measures of receptive and expressive language. The index of play diversity, or number of different actions made, was negatively related to the severity of the clinical presentation of associated autism [17].

4. ADHD

One of the most prevalent behavioral alterations associated with FXS is attentional deficit-hyperactivity disorder (ADHD). On average, among those diagnosed with FXS, 80% of males and 60% of females show symptoms of attention deficits [8]. ADHD in children with FXS is reported to be characterized by attention deficits, impulsivity, uneasiness, and fidgetiness suggestive of the ADHD inattentive sub-type; these features do not necessarily improve with age [1, 18].

Sullivan. et al., [25] gathered information from teachers and parents about ADHD symptoms based on the DSM-IV criteria in 63 children with full mutation FXS and in 56 children without disabilities based on mental age. Results from this survey suggested 60% of the boys with FXS have some type of ADHD symptoms (inattentive, hyperactive, or ADHD-combined type) when compared to the control group.

In another study with FXS boys, the investigators found the temperament and behavioral symptoms reported by the parents differed from those reported by the teachers. Additionally, data from this study suggested increased activity scores are associated with ADHD at the preschool age, and decreased smiling and laughter and elevated introversion were associated with ADHD scores. Impulsivity was strongly associated to school entry, however impulsivity in preschool had some predictive value for ADHD at the school age [19]. Other findings in FXS children with ADHD include these children having greater difficulties with auditory stimuli (compared to visual stimuli) and using an atypical processing of multimodal information [20].

Children with ADHD have difficulties in social interactions; peer rejection, social withdrawal, and negative perceptions from others are frequent consequences of ADHD. The range of these difficulties is variable from mild to severe [21]. Early detection and diagnosis of ADHD symptoms in children with FXS may be impactful in the long-term prognosis of their social functioning [22].

5. Learning Disorders

Patients with FXS can present with a wide spectrum of complications, from mild learning difficulties with a normal IQ, to mental retardation with autistic tendencies [23]. FXS is associated with slower intellectual development compared to neurotypical children, generally causing a relative drop in IQ and adaptive behavior scores. Additionally, cognitive weaknesses associated with FXS include visuospatial skills, working memory, and processing of sequential information and attention. There are also relative cognitive strengths, such as visual memory and simultaneous processing. Males tend to present with an IQ averaging 35-40 and a mental age of 5-6 years, while females can present more mildly with an average IQ of 75-80 and a wider range of intellectual involvement from normal cognition to severe impairment [24].

6. Mood Disorder

Major depressive disorder is a common comorbidity in women with the premutation FMR1, however, the data about this association is scarce and based on studies with small sample sizes and of mothers who experience higher rates of parental stress having children with FXS that may contribute to the presence of these mothers' depressive disorders. Gossett, A., et al., compared anxiety and depressive disorders in 24 women with FXS who did not have children with FXS to a cohort of 26 controls (non-carrier women). Although this study had a very small sample size, the authors reported the presence of the FXS permutation resulted in increased anxiety and depression in these mothers. Obsessive and compulsive symptoms, somatization, and interpersonal sensitivity were more frequently associated with these mothers as well [25]. Furthermore, Hunter, J.E., et al., investigated 119 adult males and 446 adult females (18-50 years old) with FXS who presented with mood and anxiety disorders as reported by their families and compared these individuals to the general population. The authors concluded repeat length was not associated with anxiety but was mildly associated with depression. Furthermore, the individuals with the premutation were at a higher risk for depression; however, the authors did conclude by indicating more evidence is needed [26].

Data was generated from the National Comorbidity Survey Replication as discussed by Bailey, R et al., where they studied 93 females with the FMR1 premutation and compared them with 2,159 women without the premutation. Their results suggested that lifetime major depressive disorder, panic disorder without agoraphobia, and current agoraphobia without panic disorder were more frequent in individuals with the FMR1 premutation sample. On the other hand, social phobia, specific phobia, post-traumatic stress disorders, and current specific phobia were less frequent in the FMR1 premutation sample. The authors further reported risk factors for depression, which included being single and having a smaller CGC repeat length. The depression was not characterized as chronic and recurrent, opposed to how depression is normally seen in the community. Having children with FXS and with behavior problems were associated with increased chance of having anxiety [27].

7. SEIZURES

Seizures and abnormalities in electroencephalogram (EEG) can be present in children between ages 2 and 9 years old who have FXS. 13% to 18% of boys with FXS have an incidence of seizures whereas approximately 5% of girls have seizures [28, 29]. Regarding the types of seizures, complex partial type is the most frequent, and partial motor and generalized seizures are less common. Seizures are more likely in those who have both FXS and ASD. Young FXS patients had age-related paroxysmal EEG patterns that resembled the ones found in the centrotemporal spikes [28].

8. SLEEP DISORDER

There is a range of 30%-90% of individuals with neurodevelopmental disorders who also present with sleep disorders [30-32]. Night walking, sleep onset delay, reduced total sleep time, and early morning waking are among the most common sleep problems in those with FXS. It is important to note that sleep disorders vary significantly across FXS disorders [33] and the current data on sleep disorders in individuals with FXS is based on limited information. Pilot data from these studies indicated that boys with FXS had difficulty falling asleep, interrupted sleep, greater variability in total sleep time, difficulty in sleep maintenance, and a dysregulated melatonin profile in comparison to age-matched controls [34, 35]. Richdale et al., [43] reported the result of sleep questionnaires completed by the parents of 13 children with FXS. 10 of them reported some sleep problems and most of them were related to more severe child psychopathology and parental stress. Obstructive sleep apnea is also associated with FXS and should be considered in differential diagnoses since it is a potential cause of psychiatric and medical problems [36].

9. MOTOR AND BEHAVIORAL DISORDERS

Restricted and repetitive behavior as well as episodes of catatonia-like attenuated behavior are likely to be evident in a minority of individuals with FXS [37]. Psychosis is seen in less than 10% of those with FXS. Catatonia can be present in FXS if it is comorbid with ADHD, ASD, IDD or any other mood disorder, but there is not enough data to support an exclusive relationship between catatonia and psychosis [6, 7].

10. AGGRESSIVE AND SELF-INJURY BEHAVIORS

Boys with FXS often present with aggressive, stereotypy, and self-injury behavior [38-40]. For example, Hess et al., [41] found in a sample of 50 male participants (8 to 24 years old) with FXS that 75% of the sample presented aggressive behaviors, 79% engaged in self-injury, and almost all of them had stereotypic behaviors. In a study by Crawford, H., et al., they found the prevalence and predictive markers of aggressive behavior in males with FXS in a longitudinal study. Similar percentages of self-injurious and aggressive behavior were found. The presence of repetitive behavior was determined to be a predictor of persistent self-injurious behavior. Impulsivity, age, and hyperactivity were associated with persistent aggressive behavior [42].

A systematic review by Hardimanand [51], found that the association of FXS with learning disabilities increases the risk of self-injury behaviors. [43] Hall et al., [52] studied compulsive and self-injury behaviors in 29 girls and 31 boys with FXS (5 to 20 years old) and found self-injury behaviors and compulsive behaviors were more commonly present in boys at 58% and 72%, compared with 17% and 55% respectively in girls.

11. OBSESSIVE-COMPULSIVE SYMPTOMS

In a study conducted by Schneider, A., et al., [53] they found 131 individuals, including 42 men and 22 women that have the FMR1 premutation with a normal neurological exam, and compared them to 48 men and 19 women as healthy age-matched controls. After completion of several neuropsychological tests and evaluations of social cognition, broad autism spectrum, and obsessive-compulsive (OC) symptoms, the study found that in males, premutation carriers showed more atypical social interaction and stereotyped behavior. On the other hand, female premutation carriers reported significantly higher rates of OC symptoms compared to the control females.

12. Discussion

Multiple genetic and environmental factors influence neuropsychiatric disorders of the general population, and these factors affect the onset and course of neuropsychiatric disorders and contribute to their complexity. The current evidence of neuropsychiatric disorders in FXS is based on studies with small sample sizes [44], however, it is unquestionable that patients with FXS frequently present with a variety of neuropsychiatric comorbidities as demonstrated from a national parent survey.[8] It is imperative to conduct early screening of these disorders in order to target potential treatments and improve the quality of the lives of FXS patients and their families. [45, 46] Since FXS patients are frequently associated with intellectual disability, the diagnosis of neuropsychiatric disorders in FXS patients is more difficult and requires substantial input from caregivers. The association of psychiatric comorbidities with seizures and learning disorders seems to appear as a cluster, and for that reason, a thorough evaluation of all these comorbidities is highly recommended. The use of behavioral checklists and semi-structured interviews can be helpful in evaluating the different behaviors and diagnosing the neuropsychiatric comorbidities [10].

Conclusion

FXS is an X-linked disorder and the most common cause of inherited intellectual disability and autism spectrum disorder. It is frequently associated with learning disabilities, attention-deficit hyperactivity disorder, and epilepsy, among other neuropsychiatric manifestations. Disorders of anxiety and social withdrawal are the core features of the FXS phenotype. The behavioral presentations range from aggression, stereotypies and self-injury behaviors. The clinical presentation of FXS is heterogeneous with clear variation depending on age, gender, and partial or full mutation. Screening for neuropsychiatric disorders is recommended. Proper diagnoses and treatments are crucial in having the best medical outcomes. While comorbidities are extensive among FXS patients, it is still difficult to fit FXS symptoms into established diagnostic categories. There are multiple powerful pharmacological treatments available, but it is necessary to understand how to utilize them, because management from a symptom-based manner can have limitations, such as unintentional aggravation of certain symptom clusters while trying to treat for another. The treatment of neuropsychiatric disorders in FXS need to be individualized and further studies on the neuropsychiatric diagnoses and medications of FXS are needed.

REFERENCES

[1] Hagerman, R. J., et al. Fragile X syndrome. *Nat. Rev. Dis. Primers*, 2017. 3: p. 17065.

[2] Verkerk, A. J., et al. Identification of a gene (FMR-1) containing a CGG repeat coincident with a breakpoint cluster region exhibiting length variation in fragile X syndrome. *Cell*, 1991. 65(5): p. 905-14.

[3] Hagerman R. J., C. A., *Fragile X Syndrome: Diagnosis, Treatment, and Research.* . 1996.

[4] Fung, L. K. and A. L. Reiss, Moving Toward Integrative, Multidimensional Research in Modern Psychiatry: Lessons Learned From Fragile X Syndrome. *Biol. Psychiatry*, 2016. 80(2): p. 100-111.

[5] Kemper, M. B., R. J. Hagerman, and D. Altshul-Stark, Cognitive profiles of boys with the fragile X syndrome. *Am. J. Med. Genet.*, 1988. 30(1-2): p. 191-200.

[6] Winarni, T. I., et al. Psychosis and catatonia in fragile X: Case report and literature review. *Intractable Rare Dis. Res.*, 2015. 4(3): p. 139-46.

[7] Keshtkarjahromi, M., et al. Psychosis and Catatonia in Fragile X Syndrome. *Cureus*, 2021. 13(1): p. e12843.

[8] Bailey, D. B., Jr., et al. Co-occurring conditions associated with FMR1 gene variations: findings from a national parent survey. *Am. J. Med. Genet. A*, 2008. 146A(16): p. 2060-9.

[9] Abbeduto, L., A. McDuffie, and A. J. Thurman, The fragile X syndrome-autism comorbidity: what do we really know? *Front. Genet.*, 2014. 5: p. 355.

[10] Thurman, A. J., et al. Psychiatric symptoms in boys with fragile X syndrome: a comparison with nonsyndromic autism spectrum disorder. *Res. Dev. Disabil.*, 2014. 35(5): p. 1072-86.

[11] Ornstein, P. A., et al. Memory skills of boys with fragile X syndrome. *Am. J. Ment. Retard,* 2008. 113(6): p. 453-65.

[12] Merenstein, S. A., et al. Molecular-clinical correlations in males with an expanded FMR1 mutation. *Am. J. Med. Genet.*, 1996. 64(2): p. 388-94.

[13] Ezell, J., et al. Prevalence and Predictors of Anxiety Disorders in Adolescent and Adult Males with Autism Spectrum Disorder and Fragile X Syndrome. *J. Autism Dev. Disord.*, 2019. 49(3): p. 1131-1141.

[14] Crawford, H., et al. Differential effects of anxiety and autism on social scene scanning in males with fragile X syndrome. *J. Neurodev. Disord.*, 2017. 9(1): p. 9.

[15] Crawford, H., et al. A Behavioural Assessment of Social Anxiety and Social Motivation in Fragile X, Cornelia de Lange and Rubinstein-Taybi Syndromes. *J. Autism Dev. Disord.*, 2020. 50(1): p. 127-144.

[16] Richards, C., et al. Prevalence of autism spectrum disorder phenomenology in genetic disorders: a systematic review and meta-analysis. *Lancet Psychiatry*, 2015. 2(10): p. 909-16.

[17] McDuffie, A., et al. Symptoms of Autism in Males with Fragile X Syndrome: A Comparison to Nonsyndromic ASD Using Current ADI-R Scores. *J. Autism Dev. Disord.*, 2015. 45(7): p. 1925-37.

[18] Hagerman, R., M. Kemper, and M. Hudson, Learning disabilities and attentional problems in boys with the fragile X syndrome. *Am. J. Dis. Child*, 1985. 139(7): p. 674-8.

[19] Grefer, M., et al. The emergence and stability of attention deficit hyperactivity disorder in boys with fragile X syndrome. *J. Intellect Disabil. Res.*, 2016. 60(2): p. 167-78.

[20] Scerif, G., et al. Attention across modalities as a longitudinal predictor of early outcomes: the case of fragile X syndrome. *J. Child Psychol. Psychiatry*, 2012. 53(6): p. 641-50.

[21] de Boo, G. M. and P. J. Prins, Social incompetence in children with ADHD: possible moderators and mediators in social-skills training. *Clin. Psychol. Rev.*, 2007. 27(1): p. 78-97.

[22] Chromik, L. C., et al. The Influence of Hyperactivity, Impulsivity, and Attention Problems on Social Functioning in Adolescents and Young Adults With Fragile X Syndrome. *J. Atten. Disord.*, 2019. 23(2): p. 181-188.

[23] Garber, K. B., J. Visootsak, and S. T. Warren, Fragile X syndrome. *Eur. J. Hum. Genet.*, 2008. 16(6): p. 666-72.

[24] Berry-Kravis, E. M., et al. Drug development for neurodevelopmental disorders: lessons learned from fragile X syndrome. *Nat. Rev. Drug Discov.*, 2018. 17(4): p. 280-299.

[25] Gossett, A., et al. Psychiatric disorders among women with the fragile X premutation without children affected by fragile X syndrome. *Am. J. Med. Genet. B Neuropsychiatr. Genet.*, 2016. 171(8): p. 1139-1147.

[26] Hunter, J. E., et al. Investigation of phenotypes associated with mood and anxiety among male and female fragile X premutation carriers. *Behav. Genet.*, 2008. 38(5): p. 493-502.

[27] Roberts, J. E., et al. Mood and anxiety disorders in females with the FMR1 premutation. *Am. J. Med. Genet. B Neuropsychiatr. Genet.*, 2009. 150B(1): p. 130-9.

[28] Musumeci, S. A., et al. Epilepsy and EEG findings in males with fragile X syndrome. *Epilepsia*, 1999. 40(8): p. 1092-9.

[29] Berry-Kravis, E., et al. Seizures in fragile X syndrome: characteristics and comorbid diagnoses. *Am. J. Intellect. Dev. Disabil.*, 2010. 115(6): p. 461-72.

[30] Angriman, M., et al. Sleep in children with neurodevelopmental disabilities. *Neuropediatrics*, 2015. 46(3): p. 199-210.
[31] Jan, J. E., et al. Neurophysiology of circadian rhythm sleep disorders of children with neurodevelopmental disabilities. *Eur. J. Paediatr. Neurol.*, 2012. 16(5): p. 403-12.
[32] Kronk, R., et al. Prevalence, nature, and correlates of sleep problems among children with fragile X syndrome based on a large scale parent survey. *Sleep*, 2010. 33(5): p. 679-87.
[33] Woodford, E. C., et al. Endogenous melatonin and sleep in individuals with Rare Genetic Neurodevelopmental Disorders (RGND): A systematic review. *Sleep Med. Rev.*, 2021. 57: p. 101433.
[34] Wirojanan, J., et al. The efficacy of melatonin for sleep problems in children with autism, fragile X syndrome, or autism and fragile X syndrome. *J. Clin. Sleep Med.*, 2009. 5(2): p. 145-50.
[35] Gould, E. L., et al. Melatonin profiles and sleep characteristics in boys with fragile X syndrome: a preliminary study. *Am. J. Med. Genet.*, 2000. 95(4): p. 307-15.
[36] Curran, C., S. Debbarma, and K. Sedky, Fragile X and Obstructive Sleep Apnea Syndrome: Case Presentation and Management Challenges. *J. Clin. Sleep Med.*, 2017. 13(1): p. 137-138.
[37] Bell, L., et al. Attenuated behaviour in Cornelia de Lange and fragile X syndromes. *J. Intellect. Disabil. Res.*, 2018. 62(6): p. 486-495.
[38] Newman, I., et al. An analysis of challenging behavior, comorbid psychopathology, and Attention-Deficit/Hyperactivity Disorder in Fragile X Syndrome. *Res. Dev. Disabil.*, 2015. 38: p. 7-17.
[39] Smith, L. E., et al. Behavioral phenotype of fragile X syndrome in adolescence and adulthood. *Am. J. Intellect. Dev. Disabil.*, 2012. 117(1): p. 1-17.
[40] Symons, F. J., et al. Self-injurious behavior and fragile X syndrome: findings from the national fragile X survey. *Am. J. Intellect. Dev. Disabil.*, 2010. 115(6): p. 473-81.
[41] Hessl, D., et al. Brief report: aggression and stereotypic behavior in males with fragile X syndrome--moderating secondary genes in a

"single gene" disorder. *J. Autism. Dev. Disord.*, 2008. 38(1): p. 184-9.

[42] Hardiman, R. L. and P. McGill, How common are challenging behaviours amongst individuals with Fragile X Syndrome? A systematic review. *Res. Dev. Disabil.*, 2018. 76: p. 99-109.

[43] Crawford, H., et al. The Persistence of Self-injurious and Aggressive Behavior in Males with Fragile X Syndrome Over 8 Years: A Longitudinal Study of Prevalence and Predictive Risk Markers. *J. Autism Dev. Disord.*, 2019. 49(7): p. 2913-2922.

[44] Farzin, F., et al. Autism spectrum disorders and attention-deficit/hyperactivity disorder in boys with the fragile X premutation. *J. Dev. Behav. Pediatr.*, 2006. 27(2 Suppl): p. S137-44.

[45] Bourgeois, J. A., et al. Lifetime prevalence of mood and anxiety disorders in fragile X premutation carriers. *J. Clin. Psychiatry*, 2011. 72(2): p. 175-82.

[46] Franke, P., et al. Genotype-phenotype relationship in female carriers of the premutation and full mutation of FMR-1. *Psychiatry Res.*, 1998. 80(2): p. 113-27.

In: Fragile X Syndrome
Editor: Fabrizio Stasolla

ISBN: 978-1-68507-572-9
© 2022 Nova Science Publishers, Inc.

Chapter 3

PHARMACOTHERAPY OF FRAGILE X SYNDROME

Maria Jimena Salcedo-Arellano[1,2,3,*]*,*
Ramkumar Aishworiya[4,5]*, Randi Hagerman*[1,2]
and Dragana Protic[6]

[1]Medical Investigation of Neurodevelopmental Disorders (MIND) Institute, University of California Davis, Sacramento, CA, USA
[2]Department of Pediatrics, UC Davis School of Medicine, Sacramento, CA, USA
[3]Department of Pathology and Laboratory Medicine, UC Davis School of Medicine, Sacramento, CA, USA
[4]Child Development Unit, Khoo Teck Puat-National University Children's Medical Institute, National University Health System, Singapore, Singapore
[5]Department of Paediatrics, Yong Loo Lin School of Medicine, National University of Singapore, Singapore, Singapore
[6]Department of Pharmacology, Clinical Pharmacology and Toxicology, Faculty of Medicine University of Belgrade, Belgrade, Serbia

---

[*] Corresponding Author's E-mail: mjsalcedo@ucdavis.edu.

ABSTRACT

Background

There is no cure for fragile X syndrome (FXS). The therapeutic approach for small children with FXS should start with behavioral intervention strategies; an early start predicts achieving best outcomes. Communication and social skills interventions should be also implemented based on individual needs. Current pharmacological treatment seeks to lessen the burden of problematic behaviors that fail to improve with psychological interventions as well as co-morbid psychiatric conditions.

Objective

In this chapter we review available pharmacotherapy backed by scientific evidence to support the treatment of psychiatric comorbidities associated with FXS as well as targeted treatments in FXS.

Methods

Data presented here were identified by literature searching. Original and review articles, case reports and textbooks in English were used. The source of literature was MEDLINE (1990-2021).

Conclusion

This chapter compiles the available medications, including mechanism of action, pediatric dosage, target behavior and common adverse effects. These medications are available clinically and have proven to be beneficial to treat challenging behaviors and common mood disorders affecting individuals with FXS. Off-label targeted treatments are promising for the improvement of various cognitive functions, language development and dysregulated behavior.

Keywords: fragile X syndrome, *FMR1* gene, pharmacotherapy, targeted treatments

1. INTRODUCTION

In general, pharmacological treatment in fragile X syndrome (FXS) implies management of different health issues, including medical, neurological, and psychiatric problems. Currently there is no cure for reversing the behavioral and learning impairments commonly found in individuals with FXS, therefore therapeutic intervention is limited to management for the improvement of individual symptoms. Commonly targeted symptoms include those of attention deficit and hyperactivity disorder (ADHD), anxiety and related problems such as sensory oversensitivity, obsessive-compulsive and perseverative behaviors, aggressive and self-injurious behaviors, social deficits and sleep disorders [1]. However, some studies have demonstrated different levels of improvement in various cognitive functions with emerging possible targeted treatments for FXS [2-4].

Our knowledge on how pharmacological agents may influence the expression of the FXS behavioral phenotype is limited to their effects on several pathways known to be disrupted in FXS. The main pathways that are dysfunctional are the gamma-aminobutyric acid (GABA) pathways, the type 5 metabotropic glutamate receptor (mGluR 5) is over-active and the cyclic adenosine monophosphate (cAMP) levels are lowered in FXS [5]. Promising drug targets could impact these pathways or involve epigenetic modulation, modulation of endocannabinoids as well as regulation of messenger RNAs (mRNAs) and proteins normally regulated by the fragile X mental retardation protein (FMRP) [3]. Levels of FMRP in individuals with FXS are correlated with the number of cytosine-guanine-guanine (CGG) repeats, the higher the number of repeats the lower the level of FMRP. In addition, levels are found to be extremely low on those individuals with a fully methylated repeat expansion. Several medications, such as sertraline, metformin, cannabidiol, acamprosate, lovastatin and minocycline, are currently available for off-label treatment of targeted neurobiological abnormalities in individuals with FXS caused by the full mutation of the fragile X mental retardation 1 (*FMR1*) gene [3].

As mentioned above, individuals with FXS show behavioral alterations, usually presenting during childhood. The most common psychiatric symptoms that are sought to improve with drug treatment in children with FXS are: ADHD, anxiety, aggressiveness, compulsive disorders and sleep problems. In addition, 50 to 60% of children with FXS are diagnosed with autism spectrum disorders (ASD) [6-8], and even though some of the abnormal molecular pathways of pathology between FXS and ASD may overlap [9], and both disorders share psychiatric features, patients with idiopathic ASD may not respond with the same efficacy to specific treatments, found to be helpful for individuals with FXS with and without comorbid ASD [10-12]. In general, individuals with FXS may have greater side effects to medications at a given dose compared to the population, hence starting at a low dose and gradual titration upwards as needed for symptom reduction is recommended [13].

In this chapter, we review the available pharmacotherapy backed by scientific evidence to support the treatment of psychiatric comorbidities associated with FXS as well as targeted treatments in FXS, based on their potential to improve the function of affected signaling pathways driving the pathology of FXS, and its implications in the clinical setting.

Data presented here were identified by literature searching. Original and review articles, case reports and textbooks in English were used. The source of literature was MEDLINE (1990-2021).

2. TREATMENT OF ADHD

Symptoms of ADHD can be problematic in up to 90% of children with FXS and become targets for pharmacological treatment, in addition to behavioral interventions and individualized therapies. To improve hyperactivity, impulsive behavior, distractibility and similar symptoms, stimulants are quite useful [1]. Studies thus far show that stimulants, at usual doses, improve symptoms of ADHD in FXS. Methylphenidate and other stimulants increase dopamine and norepinephrine at the synapse and they also modulate glycogen synthase kinase-3 β (GSK3β) activity, a negative regulator of the canonical *Wnt* signaling pathway [14], one of the overlapping dysfunctional pathways between FXS and idiopathic ASD [9]. They are the most frequently used class of medication for boys with FXS and they are thought to help in ~70% of cases, on the basis of clinical evaluations [15].

Different stimulant preparations are available based on either amphetamine or methylphenidate derivatives with short acting, immediate acting, long acting, and extended release, at appropriate dosing for each individual. Stimulants exert their action by increasing levels of dopamine and norepinephrine in the pre-frontal cortex through effects at the neurotransmitter level [16]. Both these neurotransmitters have proven benefits in improving attention, task motivation and impulse control [17]. As a class, these drugs have quick onset of action and are thus effective for targeted modulation of ADHD symptoms for acute periods of time, as clinically appropriate. Duration of action varies depending on the formulation and ranges from 4 hours (short-acting preparations) to 12 hours (extended-release preparations). These drugs are usually well tolerated in FXS, especially in children older than 5 years [18]. Most common side effects are generally minor with appetite changes and gastrointestinal (GI) symptoms with abdominal pain being the most commonly reported [19]. These typically improve after the initial period of treatment and are not clinically significant. Serious but rare adverse effects include cardiovascular events including palpitations and raised blood pressure; however, these are rare with an incidence rate for serious cardiovascular effects of 3.1 per 100,000 person years in one large population-based study [20]. Of note, several studies demonstrated no added risk of sudden cardiac-related death due to stimulants compared to the general population [21-23].

However, pharmacological treatment of ADHD symptoms in children younger than 5 years of age could raise a challenge. Stimulants may induce irritability, tantrums and other behavioral problems in these children [15]. Thus, nonstimulant medications may be helpful in this population as an alternative therapy for ADHD in young children. This includes alpha 2-adrenergic receptor agonists, clonidine and guanfacine [24]. Clonidine can be helpful for children with ADHD (especially to treat hyperactivity, overstimulation, and attention/concentration problems) who also have sleep disturbances, and sleep problems [15]. Clonidine can be used as monotherapy for preschool-aged children with ADHD symptoms and in combination with other medications for the majority of older children. Guanfacine, which is less sedating than clonidine, can also be useful for the treatment of ADHD symptoms, including hyperactivity and frustration intolerance, as well as hyperarousal in children without FXS [15, 25, 26].

Although the exact mechanism of action of these drugs is not known, they are proposed to exert their effects through the numerous alpha 2-adrenergic receptors found in the prefrontal cortex [27]. Common side effects for both drugs include sedation and reduction in blood pressure in the immediate period after commencement of treatment so the treatment should start at a low dose and gradually increase. Blood pressure can be monitored especially in the initial period after treatment commencement and after each dose increase. A dose of 0.1 mg of clonidine is equivalent to a dose of 1 mg of guanfacine, and abrupt withdrawal should be avoided for both drugs to minimise the risk of rebound hypertension [15, 28].

3. TREATMENT OF ANXIETY

Anxiety disorders are common in individuals with FXS. Between 70 to 80% can suffer from anxiety [29]. Common treatment options for relieving anxiety symptoms are selective serotonin reuptake inhibitors (SSRIs). These antidepressants are the drugs of choice for the first-line treatment of anxiety [11, 15]. One of the most common drugs used to treat anxiety in patients with FXS is sertraline. Treatment with sertraline is implemented as the symptoms emerge, often in early childhood [30]. A previous study demonstrated that SSRIs at regular doses relieved symptoms of anxiety by more than 50% [24]. In addition to sertraline, other SSRIs could also be useful in the treatment of anxiety. For example, fluoxetine can be beneficial for selective mutism, a form of anxiety found in some female and male individuals with FXS [31]. SSRIs have the potential to regulate other impairments in cognitive functioning, particularly in patients affected by FXS; they can also increase the receptiveness to and benefits of other therapies [32].

Better language development was observed in young children aged 16-60 months with FXS who received low doses of sertraline, compared to those who did not [33]. A controlled trial in children ages 2 to 6 years with FXS reported a significant benefit in the expressive language on sertraline vs placebo only on those with co-morbid ASD [11]. Some individuals (approximately 20%) may experience activation as a result of SSRIs usage. Activation symptoms derived from SSRI treatment may include restlessness, mood changes, and disinhibited behaviors, including aggression [34]. Thus, fluoxetine, as the most activating, is not the SSRI of choice for very hyperactive patients with FXS. On the other hand, it may be useful for individuals with social anxiety, autism, or selective mutism [34]. In general, SSRIs may lead to suicidal ideation among depressed adolescent patients because of activating effects, but this has never been reported in FXS, although careful monitoring of patients for mood changes or depression is justified [15].

In addition to SSRIs, other antidepressants could also be useful in managing FXS-related symptoms. Bupropion is another anti-depressant that acts via multiple mechanisms and it increases the level of both noradrenergic and dopaminergic neurotransmission via re-uptake inhibition [35]. Bupropion can be a drug of choice for symptoms of depression and anxiety especially in individuals concerned with weight gain with SSRIs; placebo-controlled trials of individuals with depression have shown that bupropion helps with weight loss [36, 37]. Apart from alleviating mood disorders, bupropion can also help with symptoms of ADHD including inattention. However, because bupropion can increase the risk of seizures, especially at higher doses, it should not be used in FXS individuals who have history of seizures [13].

Selective serotonin and norepinephrine reuptake inhibitors (SNRIs, such as duloxetine and venlafaxine) are other medications which can be used for mood disorders. Duloxetine can be especially useful in individuals with mood disorders and chronic pain as the increased norepinephrine at neurotransmitters helps with pain symptoms [38]. Tricyclic antidepressants are seldom used currently due to their potentially dangerous side effects including cardiovascular events related to cardiac conduction [39]. Benzodiazepines may be used in a single dose, on an as-needed basis, when a high level of anxiety is anticipated such as with blood draws or a dental visit; however these should not be used on a long-term basis due to the potential for addiction, sedation and memory-related problems [40].

4. TREATMENT OF AGGRESSION

Aggressiveness, self-injurious behaviors and explosive outbursts tend to become more severe with age in individuals with FXS [41]. For the management of aggression, mood instability and irritability, antipsychotic medications including atypical antipsychotics, risperidone and aripiprazole could be very helpful [15, 24]. A recent study which analyzed data from 415 individuals with FXS, presenting with symptoms of irritability, aggression, agitation, and self-injurious behaviors taken from the fragile X online registry with accessible research database (FORWARD), showed that the most utilized medications for the management of these symptoms in individuals with FXS are antipsychotics, specifically aripiprazole and risperidone (37% and 27%, respectively); sertraline was also prescribed to ~7% of the subjects included in the analysis for the treatment of these behaviors. The study found associations of severe aggressiveness requiring drug treatment with the male gender, more severe intellectual disability, high levels of anxiety and ASD comorbidity. Most of the subjects (63%) did not experience any side effects from the use of their psychopharmacologic medications [42].

Risperidone, a second-generation antipsychotic medication, is effective in modulating aggressive behavior and irritability, specifically in older male patients with FXS [24]. Its precise mechanism of action is not fully understood, but the current focus is on the ability of risperidone to inhibit the D2 dopaminergic receptors and 5-HT2A serotonergic receptors in the brain. It binds with a very high affinity to 5-HT2A receptors, approximately 10-20 fold greater than to D2 receptors [43]. In addition, risperidone is an antagonist of alpha-1, alpha-2, and histamine (H1) receptors [44]. The effectiveness of risperidone as monotherapy targeting irritability in patients with FXS in a naturalistic outpatient clinical setting was assessed in a study which included 21 male patients with FXS. Participants' mean age was 14 years (SD 8.5) at the time of risperidone treatment initiation, and the final mean dose of risperidone was 2.5 mg/day. This study confirmed previous results regarding effectiveness of risperidone in patients with FXS [45].

Similarly, aripiprazole, an atypical antipsychotic, has high overall response rate and targets multiple FXS symptoms, including anxiety, aggression, unstable mood, distractibility, concentration deficits, and other behavioral impairments [15]. Aripiprazole is a partial agonist of dopaminergic D2 and agonist of 5-HT1A receptors and antagonist of alpha adrenergic and 5-HT2A receptors [46]. Low doses of aripiprazole (2.5–5.0 mg for adolescents and lower doses for younger children, e.g., ≤1 mg at bedtime) work best for patients with FXS, because agitation is a common finding at higher doses. If agitation occurs, then the dose should be decreased [15]. A prospective 12-week open-label trial of aripiprazole in 12 individuals aged 6-25 years with FXS who were free of concomitant psychoactive drug treatment revealed that aripiprazole was generally safe and well tolerated and was associated with significant improvement in irritable behavior [47].

Other atypical antipsychotics such as olanzapine and quetiapine could also be helpful for the management of aggression in individuals with FXS [18, 24]. The most reported side effect with the use of antipsychotics is weight gain. This is an important fact to account for when treating individuals with FXS, since compulsive eating behaviors to cope with symptoms of anxiety and irritability also contribute to weight gain starting in childhood. Obesity is found in 30 – 60% of individuals with FXS, and less than 10% may present with the Prader-Willi like phenotype of FXS with severe obesity, obsessive/compulsive behaviors, delayed puberty, small genitalia, hyperphagia and lack of satiation after meals [48, 49].

5. TREATMENT OF SLEEP PROBLEMS

Sleep problems are common in individuals with FXS. Between 27 and 77% of individuals with FXS suffer sleep difficulty [50, 51]. Sleep disorders in individuals with ASD are associated with deficits of memory and learning, impaired vigilance, and severity of autistic behavior [52, 53]. The first drug of choice for sleep problems in individuals with FXS is melatonin [54]. Melatonin is an endogenous neurohormone mainly synthesized and released by the pineal gland at night under normal conditions [55]. Melatonin's primary physiological function involves regulating the circadian rhythm [56], its sleep-promoting actions are mostly caused by its feedback to the suprachiasmatic nucleus, specifically on the melatonin receptors (MT1 and MT2) [57] Treatment of sleep disorders in FXS with melatonin has shown efficacy and tolerability. Benefits are reported in longer night sleep duration, shorter sleep-onset latency, and earlier sleep-onset time [54]. The most common treatment dose of melatonin in clinical studies of sleep problems in children with neurodevelopmental disorders is between 1 and 5 mg. In addition to sleep disorders, FMRP deficiency in FXS causes the overproduction of reactive oxygen species (ROS) [58] and abnormal neuronal dendritic spines [59].

Oxidative stress induces brain dysfunction contributing to the development of psychiatric disorders in individuals with FXS and ASD; moreover, morphologically immature dendritic spines are implicated in decreased memory and learning capabilities [60]. Melatonin is a very powerful free radical scavenger and antioxidant; these beneficial properties confer protection against the development of psychiatric symptoms and processes leading to neurodegeneration. Additionally, melatonin facilitates synaptic plasticity and enhances the mechanisms underlying learning and memory [61-63]. Based on its neuroprotective, antioxidant and anti-inflammatory properties, treatment with melatonin has been postulated as therapeutical candidate for the improvement of cognitive and behavior problems in FXS [64].

Clonidine can be useful for the treatment of sleep disorders in children with FXS older than 2 years of age when treatment with melatonin has proven to be ineffective. For children with severe sleep problems refractory to melatonin and clonidine, trazodone or aripiprazole have been used with promising effectiveness [39].

6. TARGETED TREATMENT IN FRAGILE X SYNDROME

The era of new targeted treatment of FXS started decades ago. Based on results of preclinical studies in animal models of FXS which revealed potential target molecules and the efficacy of targeted treatments.

Many studies have shown defects in different neurotransmitter systems [65]. Substantial research showed increased expression of postsynaptic metabotropic glutamate receptors (mGluR) and their pathways in FXS [66, 67]. Moreover, absence of FMRP has been shown to decrease synthesis of both GABA and its receptor [68]. FMRP has also been linked to ion channels regulation through interaction with the sodium-activated potassium Slack channels. FMRP also plays an indirect role in neurotransmitter release via regulating action potentials through the large conductance Ca^{2+}-activated BK (big potassium) channel [69-72].

Additionally, the targets of FMRP are voltage-gated potassium channels Kv3.1b and Kv4.2 mRNAs [70, 73]. In addition, FMRP affects other molecules important for the process of neurogenesis, such as various growth factors and molecules involved in cell signaling. Increased expression of glycogen synthase kinase 3 beta (GSK-3β), important for both adult and embryonic neurogenesis, is demonstrated in hippocampal neurons in *FMR1* knockout mice [74]. Further, there is evidence of altered levels of matrix metalloproteinase-9 (MMP9) in *Fmr1* knockout (KO) mice models, and also in humans with FXS [75]. FMRP is also involved in the regulation of brain-derived neurotrophic factor (BDNF), and dysregulation in this pathway leads to impaired synaptic plasticity [76]. In addition, decreased FMRP leads to decreased to cAMP levels, which is crucial for membrane signaling and its altered levels are associated with ASD [77].

All the findings listed above enabled the development of targeted treatments in FXS. These potential target molecules are presented in Figure 1.

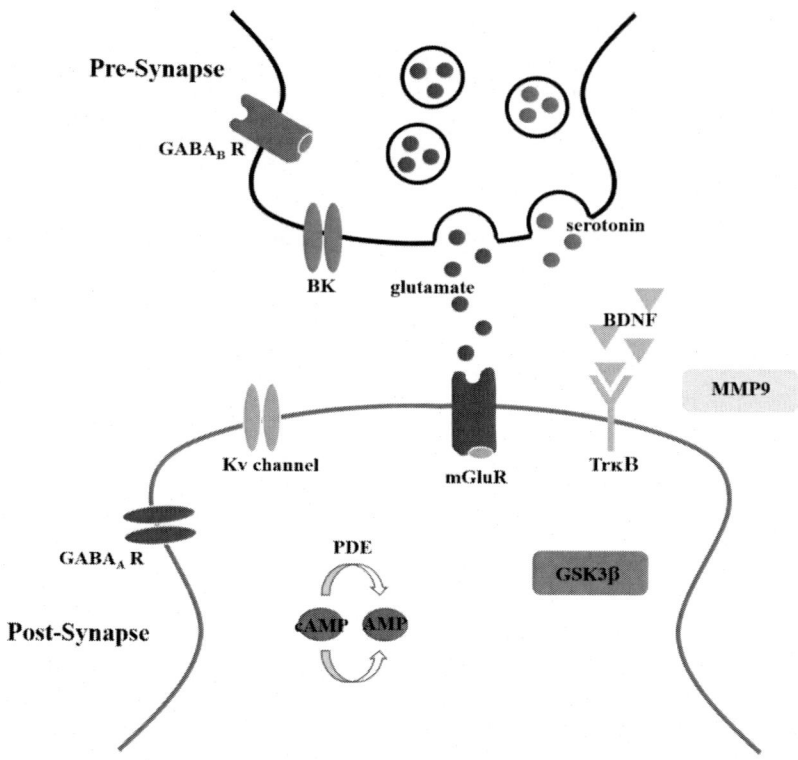

Abbreviations: GABAB R - γ-Aminobutyric acid type B receptor; BK - large conductance calcium-activated potassium channels; Kv channel - voltage-activated potassium channels; mGluR- metabotropic glutamate receptor; MMP9 - Matrix Metallopeptidase 9; BDNF - Brain-derived neurotrophic factor; TrκB - tyrosine receptor kinase B; $GABA_A$ R - γ-Aminobutyric acid type A receptor; GSK3ß - glycogen synthase kinase 3 beta; PDE – phosphodiesterase; cAMP - cyclic adenosine monophosphate; AMP - adenosine monophosphate. Adapted from Zafarullah and Tassone, 2019.

Figure 1. Potential molecular targets in Fragile X Syndrome.

The following medications have been studied for their potential therapeutic properties, anticipating the modulation or recovery of abnormal pathways translating to clinical improvement of behavior problems, learning impairments, motor or language delays and other associated medical problems, such as seizures and metabolic syndrome commonly found in individuals with FXS.

Sertraline is now often used both to treat anxiety and to enhance early development in children with FXS. Initial retrospective evaluation of treatment with low-dose sertraline (2.5 to 5.0 mg per day) for the improvement of language development in young children with FXS showed significant improvement in receptive and expressive language development. [33]. These beneficial results were further studied in a randomized controlled trial; assessments for the improvement of language development showed no significant differences between the treatment and control groups. Post hoc analysis showed that only those with FXS plus ASD demonstrated a significant benefit in the expressive language raw scores on sertraline *versus* placebo. However, sertraline showed beneficial effects in motor and visual perceptual skills and social participation in FXS patients [11, 78].

Metformin, is a biguanide antihyperglycemic medication utilized as first-line treatment for type 2 diabetes and weight loss [79]. Its mechanism of action is dependent on dose and duration of treatment. There are clear differences between acute and chronic administration of the drug. In general, metformin's mechanism of action involves AMP-activated protein kinase (AMPK)-dependent and AMPK-independent pathways [79, 80]. The efficacy of metformin as a modulator of the mGluR/mTORC1-ERK cascade in animal models of FXS was investigated in 2017. This study showed an improvement in social and cognitive behavior, as well as in morphological (dendritic spine dysgenesis and macroorchidism) and electrophysiological abnormalities (long-term depression) [78, 81]. Metformin treatment corrected circadian and cognitive deficits in the study which included the *Drosophila melanogaster* FX model [82].

Data obtained in this study documented that insulin signaling is increased in the brains of the *Drosophila melanogaster* FX model and that treatment with metformin reduced insulin signaling, leading to improvements in memory and circadian rhythm defects [82]. In the *Fmr1* KO mice model of FXS treatment with metformin showed strong inhibition of mTOR through AMPK and rescued core deficits of the phenotype [83]. The first clinical data of metformin's efficacy in FXS was obtained in 2017 when 7 patients with FXS were treated clinically for at least 6 months. Metformin was well tolerated in all patients and they had positive behavioral changes in areas such as irritability, social avoidance and aggression, as reported by caregivers; in addition to benefits in appetite and weight control in overweight patients [84]. Another report describes two adult males with FXS who showed improvement in both verbal and nonverbal IQ scores after treatment with metformin for one year [85]. They also had better performances in nonverbal and verbal tasks [85]. Metformin, after 2 years of usage, also prevented development of macroorchidism in an adolescent at age 14. This data was in correlation with data obtained in the mouse model of FXS where metformin induced the alleviation of macroorchisidm [86]. The results from the first double-blind randomized controlled trial, conducted in United States and Canada (NCT03862950, NCT03479476), evaluating the safety along with the efficacy of metformin in the treatment of language deficit and behavior problems in individuals between 6 and 40 years of age with FXS will be available by 2022. Metformin appears to be a strong candidate for a new targeted treatment for FXS [7].

Cannabidiol (CBD) is a promising treatment to address seizures and anxiety in FXS. In addition to anxiety, it could improve multiple symptoms experienced by patients with FXS [87]. Results of an open-label, multi-site clinical trial with a transdermal CBD gel (ZYN002) which included 20 children and adolescents with FXS aged between 6 and 17 years confirmed that CBD helped with anxiety in these individuals. Transdermal CBD gel was administered twice daily for 12 weeks, titrated from 50 mg to a maximum daily dose of 250 mg. The primary efficacy endpoint was change from screening to week 12 on the Anxiety, Depression, and Mood Scale (ADAMS). Treatment with CBD was well tolerated and produced clinically meaningful reductions in anxiety and behavioral symptoms in children and adolescents with FXS [87]. Results of a subsequent multicenter double blind controlled trial of the ZYN002 topical CBD preparation in over 200 children with FXS ages 3 to 18 years demonstrated that those with >90% methylation (representing 80% of the overall group) demonstrated significant improvements in the primary outcome measure, Social Avoidance on the Aberrant Behavioral Checklist fragile X version (ABC$_{FX}$) in addition to other measures (Berry-Kravis et al. 2021 under review). However, the overall group including those with mosaicism did not demonstrate efficacy. A new double blind controlled phase 3 multicenter trial is now taking place to confirm efficacy in this subgroup of FXS with >90% methylation.

Acamprosate is a medication used to maintain alcohol abstinence in patients with alcohol dependence. It may be a useful therapy for FXS. The mechanism of action is not clear, but there are suggestions that acamprosate attenuates hyper-glutamatergic states and involves ionotropic N-methyl-D-aspartate (NMDA) and metabotropic (mGluR5) glutamate receptors along with augmented intracellular calcium release and electrophysiological changes [88]. Acamprosate treatment partially or completely rescued all of the FXS phenotypes analyzed, according to dose in *Drosophila* FXS model [89]. A prospective open-label 10-week trial of acamprosate in 12 youth aged from 6 to 17 years with FXS revealed that acamprosate use at a mean dose of 1,054 ± 422 mg/day was associated with treatment response (defined by a Clinical Global Impressions Improvement (CGI-I) scale score of "very much improved" or "much improved") in 75% of subjects. Improvement was noted in social behavior and inattention/hyperactivity using multiple standard behavioral outcome measures. No changes in vital signs or significant adverse effects, including weight or laboratory measures, occurred during treatment with acamprosate. This study showed that acamprosate is generally safe and well tolerated and was associated with a significant improvement in social behavior and a reduction in inattention/ hyperactivity [90]. There is need for further controlled clinical trials to confirm its efficiency and safety in individuals with FXS.

Lovastatin is an inhibitor of the enzyme hydroxymethylglutaryl-coenzyme A (HMG-CoA) reductase used to treat hypercholesterolemia in children and adults, and reduce the risk of cardiovascular disease. Research in *Fmr1* KO mice has shown that lovastatin as an inhibitor of Ras-ERK1/2, normalized hippocampus protein synthesis [91-93]. Lovastatin corrected the excessive extra cellular receptor kinase-mediated protein synthesis and blocked mGluR5-mediated epileptiform bursting in the *Fmr1* KO hippocampal neurons, dampened the hyperexcitability seen in the visual cortex in the KO mouse and rescued the seizure phenotype in the live KO mouse [94]. Based on the positive outcome with lovastatin in *Fmr1*-/y animal models, an open-label trial tested the viability of lovastatin for the treatment of FXS in humans. A phase I study was conducted to assess the safety and efficacy of lovastatin in individuals with FXS. Fifteen patients aged between 6 and 31 years participated in the study. They were treated with escalating doses of lovastatin (up to 40 mg) for three months. The Aberrant Behavioral Checklist-Community (ABC-C) total score as primary outcome, as well as domains of the ABC_{FX} as secondary outcomes were used to assess their behavior. Lovastatin was well tolerated and minimal side effects were reported. Significant improvement was observed in the majority of the study's participants. This study showed reassuring safety data along with potential functional benefit of lovastatin in FXS [94]. Furthermore, a 20-week controlled trial of lovastatin (10 to 40 mg/day) *versus* placebo in youth with FXS, ages 10 to 17 years, combined with an open-label treatment of a parent-implemented language intervention (PILI) demonstrated significant changes in the primary outcome measures in both treatment groups [95]. The benefit attributable to treatment with lovastatin was equivalent to the benefit of those in the PILI treatment group.

Minocycline is a tetracycline antibiotic with different actions which include anti-inflammatory and anti-apoptotic effects as well as microglial clearance. It is well known that there is high plasma activity of MMP-9 in individuals with FXS.

Animal studies in the *Fmr1* KO mouse and in *Drosophila* have demonstrated that minocycline improved synaptic connections, brain structure, vocalizations, and behavior/cognition [96, 97]. Through a minocycline controlled clinical trial, MMP-9 changes in patients with FXS were observed. The results of this study suggested that activity levels of MMP-9 are lowered by minocycline in humans. In addition, this study showed that, in some cases, changes in MMP-9 activity are positively associated with improvement based on clinical measures [98]. These results are in accordance with previous results obtained in animal models [96, 97, 99]. Open-label add-on treatment trial of minocycline in FXS included 20 subjects with FXS, aged 13-32, who were randomly assigned to receive 100 mg or 200 mg of minocycline daily. The primary outcome measure was the ABC-C Irritability Subscale, and the secondary outcome measures were the other ABC-C subscales, CGI, and the visual analog scale for behavior (VAS).

Side effects were assessed using an adverse events checklist, a complete blood count (CBC), hepatic and renal function tests, and antinuclear antibody screen (ANA), done at baseline and at 8 weeks. This study confirmed significant functional benefits to FXS patients and that it is well-tolerated in those individuals [100]. A subsequent controlled trial of minocycline in children with FXS demonstrated benefits in the VAS on behavior [101] and significant improvements in habituation on event-related potential (ERP) studies for those treated with minocycline compared to controls [102]. However, patients who are treated before 8 years of age often develop darkening of the teeth and gums caused by minocycline and this side effect must be explained in detail to the family before starting treatment. Basically, metformin appears to have the same effect in lowering MMP-9 levels but without significant side effects associated with minocycline (76).

Table 1 presents a summary of the targeted treatments available, their dosage and common adverse effects.

Table 1. Available treatment for children with Fragile X syndrome

Medication	Drug class	Mechanism of action	Target problems	Dose/Day	Common side effects
Sertraline	Selective serotonin reuptake inhibitor (SSRI)	Inhibition of CNS neuronal uptake of serotonin (5HT)	Anxiety, aggressive behaviors, social participation, language development in young children	2.5 to 5.0 mg in young children (2 to 6 years) 10 to 100 mg in older children and adolescents	Diarrhea, loss of appetite, hyperhidrosis, activation (restlessness, mood changes, disinhibited behaviors), tremor
Methylphenidate	Central nervous system (CNS) stimulant	Non-competitively blocks the reuptake of dopamine and noradrenaline	Attention deficit and hyperactivity disorder (ADHD)	10 to 60 mg in children older than 6 years of age, available in extended-release presentation	Irritability, tic disorders, anxiety, insomnia, nausea, decreased appetite
Clonidine	Alpha 2-adrenergic receptor agonist	Stimulate presynaptic and postsynaptic alpha 2 adrenergic receptors in the prefrontal cortex	Hyperactivity, overstimulation, attention/concentration problems and aggression, sleep disturbances	Initial dose 0.025 mg titrate to maximum dose 0.4 mg in older children	Sedation, postural hypotension, nausea, constipation, bradycardia, xerostomia
Guanfacine	Alpha 2-adrenergic receptor agonist	Stimulate presynaptic and postsynaptic alpha 2 adrenergic receptors in the prefrontal cortex	Hyperactivity, frustration intolerance, hyperarousal	Pediatric dose: up to 1.5 mg/bid	Less sedative than clonidine, nausea, constipation, bradycardia, xerostomia
Risperidone [103]	Second-generation antipsychotic	Blocks dopamine D2 receptors in the prefrontal cortex and nucleus accumbens. Serotonin and norepinephrine reuptake inhibition	Irritability, aggression, self-injury, social impairment, stereotypical behaviors, cognition, and hyperactivity	0.5 to 3 mg based on weight. Available in long-acting injection	Weight changes, metabolic changes, and sedation. Extrapyramidal symptoms, parkinsonian features, hyperprolactinemia
Aripiprazole	Second-generation antipsychotic	Blocks dopamine D2, D3 and 5-HT1A (serotonin) receptors. Antagonist at the 5-HT2A receptor	Irritability, aggression, agitation, and self-injurious behaviors, sleep problems	5 to 15 mg	Increase in weight, somnolence (dose-response relationship) and extrapyramidal symptoms
Melatonin	Biogenic amine/endogenous hormone	Activates melatonin receptors ML1/ML2, leading to inhibition of adenylate cyclase and the cAMP signal transduction pathway; Activation of phospholipase C	Sleep disturbances	Prior to expected bedtime, starting with a low dose of 1mg increasing up to 5 mg as needed	Day-time drowsiness, headache and dizziness, transient depressive symptoms, mild tremor, mild anxiety, abdominal cramps, irritability, reduced alertness, confusion, nausea, vomiting, and hypotension

Medication	Drug class	Mechanism of action	Target problems	Dose/Day	Common side effects
Metformin	Biguanide anti-hyperglycemic	Metformin is a medication that acts through the AMP-activated protein kinase (AMPK) pathway, which then impacts both the mTOR and ERK/MAPK pathways. Decreases the level of protein MMP-9 in FXS	Cognitive abilities, language, weight management	1000 mg < 50kg 2000 mg > 50kg available in extended-release	Nausea, diarrhea, headache, gas, weight loss, dizziness, inadequate vitamin B12
Minocycline	Tetracycline antibiotic, considered a neuroprotective agent	Multiple mechanisms of action including anti-inflammatory, MMP inhibition and anti-apoptotic effects. Inhibition of activity of the protein MMP-9 in FXS	Overall clinical improvement, anxiety and other mood-related behaviors	25 mg < 25 kg 50 mg 25-45 kg 100 mg > 45 mg	Nausea, headache, diarrhea, dizziness, loss of appetite, oral cavity and tooth discoloration
Acamprosate	Synthetic amino acid, structural analogue of the neurotransmitter γ-aminobutyric acid (GABA)	mGluR5 receptor antagonist	Anxiety, social behavior, hyperactivity, alcohol dependence[104]	1332 mg < 50 kg 1998 mg > 50 kg	Irritability, depression, GI symptoms (constipation, diarrhea)
Cannabidiol	Non-euphoric exogenous phyto cannabinoid in cannabis	Multiple: Interact with an FXS-compromised endocannabinoid system; positively affect synaptic plasticity; a positive allosteric modulator of GABAA receptors; Serotonin 1A receptors modulator	Reductions in social avoidance and anxiety, as well as improvements in sleep, feeding, motor coordination, language skills, anxiety, seizures and sensory processing	Oral tincture.25 to 50 mg per dose up to bid Topical ointments: 125 mg to 500 mg bid	Sedation, but rare cases of activation. Higher doses may cause liver function test elevations. Topicals may cause skin rash or irritation

CONCLUSION

Considering the significant progress in the field of pharmacology in FXS made over the past 2 decades, we are entering a new era in the pharmacotherapeutic approach to treatments for patients with FXS. Animal models continue to provide new information on the abnormal processes leading to pathology and the clinical phenotype of FXS. New compounds and non-FDA approved medications are currently under investigation for their potential benefits to target specific deficits in FXS. These include mavoglurant (AFQ056), AZD7325 (NCT03140813), trofinetide and gaboxadol (OV101) (NCT03697161). The recent news that BPN14770, a phosphodiesterase 4D (PDE4D) inhibitor that inhibits the metabolism of cAMP which is too low in FXS, can improve cognition as measured by the NIH toolbox in 30 adults with FXS excited many investigators and family members because no previous medication has improved cognition in adults with FXS [4]. Currently further phase 3 controlled trials are taking place with this PDE4D inhibitor.

We reviewed the medications that have shown efficacy for the treatment of psychiatric morbidities commonly associated with FXS, we also identified recently studied targeted treatments that are available clinically and can be prescribed for patients with FXS. Many of these medications can also be used simultaneously, although only one medication should be added at a time to facilitate an analysis of its efficacy. Since many overlapping pathways and proteins are disrupted in the absence of FMRP, it is likely that a combination of medications will be beneficial in those with FXS. Physicians should be encouraged to utilize targeted treatments for the improvement of learning and language abilities as well as behavioral improvements in FXS as they become available clinically. These new medications will not only improve the symptoms in individuals with FXS but may have the potential to increase their level of independence and cognition over time. For those individuals starting such treatments early in life, long-term follow-up studies will hopefully show reversal of many of the symptoms of FXS. Effective management of the comorbid conditions associated with FXS will also be important to ensure optimal quality of life for individuals with FXS and their families.

REFERENCES

[1] Berry-Kravis, E; Sumis, A; Hervey, C; Mathur, S. Clinic-based retrospective analysis of psychopharmacology for behavior in fragile x syndrome. *Int J Pediatr.*, 2012, 2012, 843016.

[2] Lee, AW; Ventola, P; Budimirovic, D; Berry-Kravis, E; Visootsak, J. Clinical Development of Targeted Fragile X Syndrome Treatments: An Industry Perspective. *Brain Sci.*, 2018, 8(12).

[3] Protic, D; Salcedo-Arellano, MJ; Dy, JB; Potter, LA; Hagerman, RJ. New Targeted Treatments for Fragile X Syndrome. *Curr Pediatr Rev.*, 2019, 15(4), 251-8.

[4] Berry-Kravis, EM; Harnett, MD; Reines, SA; Reese, MA; Ethridge, LE; Outterson, AH; et al. Inhibition of phosphodiesterase-4D in adults with fragile X syndrome: a randomized, placebo-controlled, phase 2 clinical trial. *Nat Med.*. 2021, 27(5), 862-70.

[5] Hagerman, RJ; Hagerman, PJ. Fragile X Syndrome: Lessons Learned and What New Treatment Avenues Are on the Horizon. *Annu Rev Pharmacol Toxicol.*, 2021.

[6] Harris, SW; Hessl, D; Goodlin-Jones, B; Ferranti, J; Bacalman, S; Barbato, I; et al. Autism profiles of males with fragile X syndrome. *Am J Ment Retard.*, 2008, 113(6), 427-38.

[7] Hatton, DD; Sideris, J; Skinner, M; Mankowski, J; Bailey, DB; Jr. Roberts, J; et al. Autistic behavior in children with fragile X syndrome: prevalence, stability, and the impact of FMRP. *Am J Med Genet A.*, 2006, 140A(17), 1804-13.

[8] Roberts, JE; Weisenfeld, LA; Hatton, DD; Heath, M; Kaufmann, WE. Social approach and autistic behavior in children with fragile X syndrome. *J Autism Dev Disord.*, 2007, 37(9), 1748-60.

[9] Salcedo-Arellano, MJ; Cabal-Herrera, AM; Punatar, RH; Clark, CJ; Romney, CA; Hagerman, RJ. Overlapping Molecular Pathways

Leading to Autism Spectrum Disorders, Fragile X Syndrome, and Targeted Treatments. *Neurotherapeutics.*, 2020.

[10] Potter, LA; Scholze, DA; Biag, HMB; Schneider, A; Chen, Y; Nguyen, DV; et al. A Randomized Controlled Trial of Sertraline in Young Children With Autism Spectrum Disorder. *Front Psychiatry.*, 2019, 10, 810.

[11] Greiss, Hess, L; Fitzpatrick, SE; Nguyen, DV; Chen, Y; Gaul, KN; Schneider, A; et al. A Randomized, Double-Blind, Placebo-Controlled Trial of Low-Dose Sertraline in Young Children With Fragile X Syndrome. *J Dev Behav Pediatr.*, 2016, 37(8), 619-28.

[12] Rajaratnam, A; Potter, LA; Biag, HMB; Schneider, A; Petrasic, IC; Hagerman, RJ. Review of Autism Profiles and Response to Sertraline in Fragile X Syndrome-Associated Autism vs. Non-syndromic Autism: Next Steps for Targeted Treatment. *Front Neurol.*, 2020, 11, 581429.

[13] Hagerman, RJ; Protic, D; Berry-Kravis, E. Medical, Psychopharmacological, and Targeted Treatment for FXS. In: Hagerman RJ, Hagerman PJ, editors. *Fragile X Syndrome and Premutation Disorders*. London: Mac Keith Press, 2020. p. 41-59.

[14] Beurel, E; Grieco, SF; Jope, RS. Glycogen synthase kinase-3 (GSK3): regulation, actions, and diseases. *Pharmacol Ther.*, 2015, 148, 114-31.

[15] Hagerman, RJ; Berry-Kravis, E; Kaufmann, WE; Ono, MY; Tartaglia, N; Lachiewicz, A; et al. Advances in the treatment of fragile X syndrome. *Pediatrics.*, 2009, 123(1), 378-90.

[16] Brown, KA; Samuel, S; Patel, DR. Pharmacologic management of attention deficit hyperactivity disorder in children and adolescents: a review for practitioners. *Transl Pediatr.*, 2018, 7(1), 36-47.

[17] Arnsten, AFT; Berridge, CW; Adler, LA; Spencer, TJ; Wilens, TE. Catecholamine influences on prefrontal cortex circuits and function. *Attention-Deficit Hyperactivity Disorder in Adults and Children*, 2015. p. 161-73.

[18] Hagerman, RJ; Polussa, J. Treatment of the psychiatric problems associated with fragile X syndrome. *Curr Opin Psychiatry.*, 2015, 28(2), 107-12.

[19] Markowitz, JS; Straughn, AB; Patrick, KS. Advances in the pharmacotherapy of attention-deficit-hyperactivity disorder: focus on methylphenidate formulations. *Pharmacotherapy.*, 2003, 23(10), 1281-99.

[20] Cooper, WO; Habel, LA; Sox, CM; Chan, KA; Arbogast, PG; Cheetham, TC; et al. ADHD drugs and serious cardiovascular events in children and young adults. *N Engl J Med.*, 2011, 365(20), 1896-904.

[21] Olfson, M; Huang, C; Gerhard, T; Winterstein, AG; Crystal, S; Allison, PD; et al. Stimulants and cardiovascular events in youth with attention-deficit/hyperactivity disorder. *J Am Acad Child Adolesc Psychiatry.*, 2012, 51(2), 147-56.

[22] Schelleman, H; Bilker, WB; Strom, BL; Kimmel, SE; Newcomb, C; Guevara, JP; et al. Cardiovascular events and death in children exposed and unexposed to ADHD agents. *Pediatrics.*, 2011, 127(6), 1102-10.

[23] Dalsgaard, S; Kvist, AP; Leckman, JF; Nielsen, HS; Simonsen, M. Cardiovascular safety of stimulants in children with attention-deficit/hyperactivity disorder: a nationwide prospective cohort study. *J Child Adolesc Psychopharmacol.*, 2014, 24(6), 302-10.

[24] Berry-Kravis, E; Potanos, K. Psychopharmacology in fragile X syndrome--present and future. *Ment Retard Dev Disabil Res Rev.*, 2004, 10(1), 42-8.

[25] Hunt, RD; Arnsten, AF; Asbell, MD. An open trial of guanfacine in the treatment of attention-deficit hyperactivity disorder. *J Am Acad Child Adolesc Psychiatry.*, 1995, 34(1), 50-4.

[26] Scahill, L; Chappell, PB; Kim, YS; Schultz, RT; Katsovich, L; Shepherd, E; et al. A placebo-controlled study of guanfacine in the treatment of children with tic disorders and attention deficit hyperactivity disorder. *Am J Psychiatry.*, 2001, 158(7), 1067-74.

[27] Jain, R; Segal, S; Kollins, SH; Khayrallah, M. Clonidine extended-release tablets for pediatric patients with attention-deficit/hyperactivity disorder. *J Am Acad Child Adolesc Psychiatry.*, 2011, 50(2), 171-9.

[28] Newcorn, JH; Schulz, K; Harrison, M; DeBellis, MD; Udarbe, JK; Halperin, JM. α2 Adrenergic Agonists. *Pediatric Clinics of North America.*, 1998, 45(5), 1099-122.

[29] Ballinger, EC; Cordeiro, L; Chavez, AD; Hagerman, RJ; Hessl, D. Emotion potentiated startle in fragile X syndrome. *J Autism Dev Disord.*, 2014, 44(10), 2536-46.

[30] Hanson, AC; Hagerman, RJ. Serotonin dysregulation in Fragile X Syndrome: implications for treatment. *Intractable Rare Dis Res.*, 2014, 3(4), 110-7.

[31] Hagerman, RJ; Hills, J; Scharfenaker, S; Lewis, H. Fragile X syndrome and selective mutism. *Am J Med Genet.*, 1999, 83(4), 313-7.

[32] Murphy, TK; Bengtson, MA; Tan, JY; Carbonell, E; Levin, GM. Selective serotonin reuptake inhibitors in the treatment of paediatric anxiety disorders: a review. *Int Clin Psychopharmacol.*, 2000, 15 Suppl 2, S47-63.

[33] Winarni, TI; Schneider, A; Borodyanskara, M; Hagerman, RJ. Early intervention combined with targeted treatment promotes cognitive and behavioral improvements in young children with fragile x syndrome. *Case Rep Genet.*, 2012, 2012, 280813.

[34] Hagerman, RJ; Fulton, MJ; Leaman, A; Riddle, J; Hagerman, K; Sobesky, W. A survey of fluoxetine therapy in fragile X syndrome. *Developmental brain dysfunction.*, 1994, 7, 155-64.

[35] Fava, M; Rush, AJ; Thase, ME; Clayton, A; Stahl, SM; Pradko, JF; et al. 15 years of clinical experience with bupropion HCl: from bupropion to bupropion SR to bupropion XL. *Prim Care Companion J Clin Psychiatry.*, 2005, 7(3), 106-13.

[36] Jain, AK; Kaplan, RA; Gadde, KM; Wadden, TA; Allison, DB; Brewer, ER; et al. Bupropion SR vs. placebo for weight loss in obese

patients with depressive symptoms. *Obes Res.*, 2002, 10(10), 1049-56.

[37] Anderson, JW; Greenway, FL; Fujioka, K; Gadde, KM; McKenney, J; O'Neil, PM. Bupropion SR enhances weight loss: a 48-week double-blind, placebo- controlled trial. *Obes Res.*, 2002, 10(7), 633-41.

[38] Shelton, RC. Serotonin and Norepinephrine Reuptake Inhibitors. *Handb Exp Pharmacol.*, 2019, 250, 145-80.

[39] Hagerman, RJ; Protic, D; Berry-Kravis, E. In: Hagerman RJ, Hagerman PJ, editors. *Fragile X Syndrome and Premutation Disorders*. London: Mac Keith Press, 2020. p. 41-59.

[40] Bandelow, B; Michaelis, S; Wedekind, D. Treatment of anxiety disorders. *Dialogues in Clinical Neuroscience.*, 2017, 19(2), 93-107.

[41] Tsiouris, JA; Brown, WT. Neuropsychiatric symptoms of fragile X syndrome: pathophysiology and *pharmacotherapy.*, CNS Drugs. 2004, 18(11), 687-703.

[42] Eckert, EM; Dominick, KC; Pedapati, EV; Wink, LK; Shaffer, RC; Andrews, H; et al. Pharmacologic Interventions for Irritability, Aggression, Agitation and Self-Injurious Behavior in Fragile X Syndrome: An Initial Cross-Sectional Analysis. *J Autism Dev Disord.*, 2019, 49(11), 4595-602.

[43] Fenton, C; Scott, LJ. Risperidone: a review of its use in the treatment of bipolar mania. *CNS Drugs.*, 2005, 19(5), 429-44.

[44] Marder, SR; Meibach, RC. Risperidone in the treatment of schizophrenia. *Am J Psychiatry.*, 1994, 151(6), 825-35.

[45] Dominick, KC; Wink, LK; Pedapati, EV; Shaffer, R; Sweeney, JA; Erickson, CA. Risperidone Treatment for Irritability in Fragile X Syndrome. *J Child Adolesc Psychopharmacol.*, 2018, 28(4), 274-8.

[46] Nasrallah, HA. Atypical antipsychotic-induced metabolic side effects: insights from receptor-binding profiles. *Mol Psychiatry.*, 2008, 13(1), 27-35.

[47] Erickson, CA; Stigler, KA; Wink, LK; Mullett, JE; Kohn, A; Posey, DJ; et al. A prospective open-label study of aripiprazole in fragile X syndrome. *Psychopharmacology (Berl).*, 2011, 216(1), 85-90.

[48] McLennan, Y; Polussa, J; Tassone, F; Hagerman, R. Fragile x syndrome. *Curr Genomics.*, 2011, 12(3), 216-24.

[49] Nowicki, ST; Tassone, F; Ono, MY; Ferranti, J; Croquette, MF; Goodlin-Jones, B; et al. The Prader-Willi phenotype of fragile X syndrome. *J Dev Behav Pediatr.*, 2007, 28(2), 133-8.

[50] Kronk, R; Dahl, R; Noll, R. Caregiver reports of sleep problems on a convenience sample of children with fragile X syndrome. *Am J Intellect Dev Disabil.*, 2009, 114(6), 383-92.

[51] Richdale, AL. Sleep problems in autism: prevalence, cause, and intervention. *Dev Med Child Neurol.*, 1999, 41(1), 60-6.

[52] Mazurek, MO; Sohl, K. Sleep and Behavioral Problems in Children with Autism Spectrum Disorder. *J Autism Dev Disord.*, 2016, 46(6), 1906-15.

[53] Wiggs, L; Stores, G. Severe sleep disturbance and daytime challenging behaviour in children with severe learning disabilities. *J Intellect Disabil Res.*, 1996, 40 (Pt 6), 518-28.

[54] Wirojanan, J; Jacquemont, S; Diaz, R; Bacalman, S; Anders, TF; Hagerman, RJ; et al. The efficacy of melatonin for sleep problems in children with autism, fragile X syndrome, or autism and fragile X syndrome. *J Clin Sleep Med.*, 2009, 5(2), 145-50.

[55] Reiter, RJ; Calvo, JR; Karbownik, M; Qi, W; Tan, DX. Melatonin and its relation to the immune system and inflammation. *Ann N Y Acad Sci.*, 2000, 917, 376-86.

[56] Foulkes, NS; assone-Corsi, P; Borjigin, J; Snyder, SH; Snyder, SH. Rhythmic transcription: the molecular basis of circadian melatonin synthesis. *Trends in Neurosciences.*, 1997, 20(10), 487-92.

[57] Srinivasan, V; Pandi-Perumal, SR; Trahkt, I; Spence, DW; Poeggeler, B; Hardeland, R; et al. Melatonin and melatonergic drugs on sleep: possible mechanisms of action. *Int J Neurosci.*, 2009, 119(6), 821-46.

[58] el Bekay, R; Romero-Zerbo, Y; Decara, J; Sanchez-Salido, L; Del, Arco-Herrera, I; Rodriguez-de, Fonseca, F; et al. Enhanced markers of oxidative stress, altered antioxidants and NADPH-oxidase activation in brains from Fragile X mental retardation 1-deficient

mice, a pathological model for Fragile X syndrome. *Eur J Neurosci.*, 2007, 26(11), 3169-80.

[59] Nimchinsky, EA; Oberlander, AM; Svoboda, K. Abnormal Development of Dendritic Spines inFMR1Knock-Out Mice. *The Journal of Neuroscience.*, 2001, 21(14), 5139-46.

[60] Kasai, H; Fukuda, M; Watanabe, S; Hayashi-Takagi, A; Noguchi, J. Structural dynamics of dendritic spines in memory and cognition. *Trends Neurosci.*, 2010, 33(3), 121-9.

[61] El-Sherif, Y; Tesoriero, J; Hogan, MV; Wieraszko, A. Melatonin regulates neuronal plasticity in the hippocampus. *J Neurosci Res.*, 2003, 72(4), 454-60.

[62] Baydas, G; Ozer, M; Yasar, A; Tuzcu, M; Koz, ST. Melatonin improves learning and memory performances impaired by hyperhomocysteinemia in rats. *Brain Res.*, 2005, 1046(1-2), 187-94.

[63] Baydas, G; Ozveren, F; Akdemir, I; Tuzcu, M; Yasar, A. Learning and memory deficits in rats induced by chronic thinner exposure are reversed by melatonin. *J Pineal Res.*, 2005, 39(1), 50-6.

[64] Won, J; Jin, Y; Choi, J; Park, S; Lee, TH; Lee, SR; et al. Melatonin as a Novel Interventional Candidate for Fragile X Syndrome with Autism Spectrum Disorder in Humans. *Int J Mol Sci.*, 2017, 18(6).

[65] Zafarullah, M; Tassone, F. Molecular Biomarkers in Fragile X Syndrome. *Brain Sci.*, 2019, 9(5).

[66] Gross, C; Hoffmann, A; Bassell, GJ; Berry-Kravis, EM. Therapeutic Strategies in Fragile X Syndrome: From Bench to Bedside and Back. *Neurotherapeutics.*, 2015, 12(3), 584-608.

[67] Ligsay, A; Hagerman, RJ. Review of targeted treatments in fragile X syndrome. *Intractable Rare Dis Res.*, 2016, 5(3), 158-67.

[68] Braat, S; D'Hulst, C; Heulens, I; De, Rubeis, S; Mientjes, E; Nelson, DL; et al. The GABAA receptor is an FMRP target with therapeutic potential in fragile X syndrome. *Cell Cycle.*, 2015, 14(18), 2985-95.

[69] Salcedo-Arellano, MJ; Hagerman, RJ; Martinez-Cerdeno, V. Fragile X syndrome: clinical presentation, pathology and treatment. *Gac Med Mex.*, 2020, 156(1), 60-6.

[70] Ferron, L. Fragile X mental retardation protein controls ion channel expression and activity. *J Physiol.*, 2016, 594(20), 5861-7.

[71] Deng, PY; Rotman, Z; Blundon, JA; Cho, Y; Cui, J; Cavalli, V; et al. FMRP regulates neurotransmitter release and synaptic information transmission by modulating action potential duration via BK channels. *Neuron.*, 2013, 77(4), 696-711.

[72] Brown, MR; Kronengold, J; Gazula, VR; Chen, Y; Strumbos, JG; Sigworth, FJ; et al. Fragile X mental retardation protein controls gating of the sodium-activated potassium channel Slack. *Nat Neurosci.*, 2010, 13(7), 819-21.

[73] Darnell, JC; Van, Driesche, SJ; Zhang, C; Hung, KY; Mele, A; Fraser, CE; et al. FMRP stalls ribosomal translocation on mRNAs linked to synaptic function and autism. *Cell.*, 2011, 146(2), 247-61.

[74] Portis, S; Giunta, B; Obregon, D; Tan, J. The role of glycogen synthase kinase-3 signaling in neurodevelopment and fragile X syndrome. *Int J Physiol Pathophysiol Pharmacol.*, 2012, 4(3), 140-8.

[75] Jasoliya, M; Bowling, H; Petrasic, IC; Durbin-Johnson, B; Klann, E; Bhattacharya, A; et al. Blood-Based Biomarkers Predictive of Metformin Target Engagement in Fragile X Syndrome. *Brain Science.*, 2020, 10(6), 361.

[76] Louhivuori, LM; Jansson, L; Turunen, PM; Jantti, MH; Nordstrom, T; Louhivuori, V; et al. Transient receptor potential channels and their role in modulating radial glial-neuronal interaction: a signaling pathway involving mGluR5. *Stem Cells Dev.*, 2015, 24(6), 701-13.

[77] Choi, CH; Schoenfeld, BP; Weisz, ED; Bell, AJ; Chambers, DB; Hinchey, J; et al. PDE-4 inhibition rescues aberrant synaptic plasticity in Drosophila and mouse models of fragile X syndrome. *J Neurosci.*, 2015, 35(1), 396-408.

[78] Salcedo-Arellano, MJ; Dufour, B; McLennan, Y; Martinez-Cerdeno, V; Hagerman, R. Fragile X syndrome and associated disorders: Clinical aspects and pathology. *Neurobiol Dis.*, 2020, 136, 104740.

[79] Romero, R; Erez, O; Huttemann, M; Maymon, E; Panaitescu, B; Conde-Agudelo, A; et al. Metformin, the aspirin of the 21st century:

its role in gestational diabetes mellitus, prevention of preeclampsia and cancer, and the promotion of longevity. *Am J Obstet Gynecol.*, 2017, 217(3), 282-302.

[80] Viollet, B; Guigas, B; Sanz, Garcia, N; Leclerc, J; Foretz, M; Andreelli, F. Cellular and molecular mechanisms of metformin: an overview. *Clin Sci (Lond).*, 2012, 122(6), 253-70.

[81] Wang, Y; Zhao, J; Guo, FL; Gao, X; Xie, X; Liu, S; et al. Metformin Ameliorates Synaptic Defects in a Mouse Model of AD by Inhibiting Cdk5 Activity. *Front Cell Neurosci.*, 2020, 14, 170.

[82] Monyak, RE; Emerson, D; Schoenfeld, BP; Zheng, X; Chambers, DB; Rosenfelt, C; et al. Insulin signaling misregulation underlies circadian and cognitive deficits in a Drosophila fragile X model. *Mol Psychiatry.*, 2017, 22(8), 1140-8.

[83] Gantois, I; Popic, J; Khoutorsky, A; Sonenberg, N. Metformin for Treatment of Fragile X Syndrome and Other Neurological Disorders. *Annu Rev Med.*, 2019, 70, 167-81.

[84] Dy, ABC; Tassone, F; Eldeeb, M; Salcedo-Arellano, MJ; Tartaglia, N; Hagerman, R. Metformin as targeted treatment in fragile X syndrome. *Clin Genet.*, 2018, 93(2), 216-22.

[85] Protic, D; Aydin, EY; Tassone, F; Tan, MM; Hagerman, RJ; Schneider, A. Cognitive and behavioral improvement in adults with fragile X syndrome treated with metformin-two cases. *Mol Genet Genomic Med.*, 2019, 7(7), e00745.

[86] Protic, D; Kaluzhny, P; Tassone, F; Hagerman, R. Prepubertal Metformin Treatment in Fragile X Syndrome Alleviated Macroorchidism: A Case Study. *Advances in Clinical and Translational Research.*, 2019, 3(1), 1-5.

[87] Heussler, H; Cohen, J; Silove, N; Tich, N; Bonn-Miller, MO; Du, W; et al. A phase 1/2, open-label assessment of the safety, tolerability, and efficacy of transdermal cannabidiol (ZYN002) for the treatment of pediatric fragile X syndrome. *J Neurodev Disord.*, 2019, 11(1), 16.

[88] Mann, K; Kiefer, F; Spanagel, R; Littleton, J. Acamprosate: recent findings and future research directions. *Alcohol Clin Exp Res.*, 2008, 32(7), 1105-10.

[89] Hutson, RL; Thompson, RL; Bantel, AP; Tessier, CR. Acamprosate rescues neuronal defects in the Drosophila model of Fragile X Syndrome. *Life Sci.*, 2018, 195, 65-70.

[90] Erickson, CA; Wink, LK; Ray, B; Early, MC; Stiegelmeyer, E; Mathieu-Frasier, L; et al. Impact of acamprosate on behavior and brain-derived neurotrophic factor: an open-label study in youth with fragile X syndrome. *Psychopharmacology (Berl).*, 2013, 228(1), 75-84.

[91] Osterweil, EK; Chuang, SC; Chubykin, AA; Sidorov, M; Bianchi, R; Wong, RK; et al. Lovastatin corrects excess protein synthesis and prevents epileptogenesis in a mouse model of fragile X syndrome. *Neuron.*, 2013, 77(2), 243-50.

[92] Schafer, WR; Kim, R; Sterne, R; Thorner, J; Kim, SH; Rine, J. Genetic and pharmacological suppression of oncogenic mutations in ras genes of yeast and humans. *Science.*, 1989, 245(4916), 379-85.

[93] Mendola, CE; Backer, JM. Lovastatin blocks N-ras oncogene-induced neuronal differentiation. *Cell Growth Differ.*, 1990, 1(10), 499-502.

[94] Caku, A; Pellerin, D; Bouvier, P; Riou, E; Corbin, F. Effect of lovastatin on behavior in children and adults with fragile X syndrome: an open-label study. *Am J Med Genet A.*, 2014, 164A(11), 2834-42.

[95] Thurman, AJ; Potter, LA; Kim, K; Tassone, F; Banasik, A; Potter, SN; et al. Controlled trial of lovastatin combined with an open-label treatment of a parent-implemented language intervention in youth with fragile X syndrome. *J Neurodev Disord.*, 2020, 12(1), 12.

[96] Siller, SS; Broadie, K. Neural circuit architecture defects in a Drosophila model of Fragile X syndrome are alleviated by minocycline treatment and genetic removal of matrix metalloproteinase. *Dis Model Mech.*, 2011, 4(5), 673-85.

[97] Bilousova, TV; Dansie, L; Ngo, M; Aye, J; Charles, JR; Ethell, DW; et al. Minocycline promotes dendritic spine maturation and improves behavioural performance in the fragile X mouse model. *J Med Genet.*, 2009, 46(2), 94-102.

[98] Dziembowska, M; Pretto, DI; Janusz, A; Kaczmarek, L; Leigh, MJ; Gabriel, N; et al. High MMP-9 activity levels in fragile X syndrome are lowered by minocycline. *Am J Med Genet A.*, 2013, 161A(8), 1897-903.

[99] Toledo, MA; Wen, TH; Binder, DK; Ethell, IM; Razak, KA. Reversal of ultrasonic vocalization deficits in a mouse model of Fragile X Syndrome with minocycline treatment or genetic reduction of MMP-9. *Behav Brain Res.*, 2019, 372, 112068.

[100] Paribello, C; Tao, L; Folino, A; Berry-Kravis, E; Tranfaglia, M; Ethell, IM; et al. Open-label add-on treatment trial of minocycline in fragile X syndrome. *BMC Neurol.*, 2010, 10, 91.

[101] Leigh, MJ; Nguyen, DV; Mu, Y; Winarni, TI; Schneider, A; Chechi, T; et al. A randomized double-blind, placebo-controlled trial of minocycline in children and adolescents with fragile x syndrome. *J Dev Behav Pediatr.*, 2013, 34(3), 147-55.

[102] Schneider, A; Leigh, MJ; Adams, P; Nanakul, R; Chechi, T; Olichney, J; et al. Electrocortical changes associated with minocycline treatment in fragile X syndrome. *J Psychopharmacol.*, 2013, 27(10), 956-63.

[103] McNeil, SE; Gibbons, JR; Cogburn, M. *Risperidone: StatPearls Publishing LLC.*; 2021 [updated August 9, 2021. Available from: https: //www.ncbi.nlm.nih.gov/books/NBK459313/.

[104] Salcedo-Arellano, MJ; Lozano, R; Tassone, F; Hagerman, RJ; Saldarriaga, W. Alcohol use dependence in fragile X syndrome. *Intractable Rare Dis Res.*, 2016, 5(3), 207-13.

In: Fragile X Syndrome
Editor: Fabrizio Stasolla

ISBN: 978-1-68507-572-9
© 2022 Nova Science Publishers, Inc.

Chapter 4

GENERAL FEATURES AND CONCEPTUAL ISSUES ON FRAGILE X SYNDROME

Donatella Ciarmoli[*] *and Fabrizio Stasolla*
"Giustino Fortunato" University of Benevento, Italy

ABSTRACT

Background

Fragile X syndrome (FXS) is a rare genetic disorder resulting from the mutation of the FMR1 gene on the X chromosome. The syndrome is characterized by learning difficulties, social isolation, stereotyped behaviors, communication impairments, intellectual deficits, and is frequently associated with anxiety, avoidance, impulsivity, hyperactivity and seizures.

---

[*] Corresponding Author's E-mail: d.ciarmoli1@studenti.unifortunato.eu.

Objectives

This chapter aims to address the various issues related to the fragile x syndrome from a conceptual point of view in order to have an exhaustive overview.

Method

Empirical contributions were selected through a systematic search.

Results

A comprehensive overview of the FXS was provided.

Conclusion

FXS is a complex genetic disorder which requires specific combined interventions.

Keywords: fragile x syndrome, brain structure, treatments, social communication, intellectual development, challenging behavior

1. INTRODUCTION

Fragile X syndrome (FXS) is a genetic disorder due to an excessive length regarding a repetitive sequence of trinucleotides (CGG) in the FMR1 gene, located on the long arm of X chromosome [1-2-3]. The FXS represents one of the frequent causes of severe to profound developmental disabilities. Consequently, a wide range of intellectual disabilities, learning difficulties, anxiety, attention deficits, impulsivity, and autistic-like behaviors are commonly observed. Additionally, self-injury, aggression, and disruptive behavior usually emerge. Hand biting and flapping related stereotypic behaviors are described as part of the phenotype [4].

Accordingly, individuals with FXS may be passive and isolated, have poor independence and constantly rely on caregivers' assistance, and may have negative outcomes on their quality of life [5].

Children with severe to profound developmental and/or multiple disabilities (i.e., a combination of intellectual, motor, and sensorial disabilities) may pose serious problems to parents, staff, and caregivers within home, educational, medical, and rehabilitative settings. In fact, they are often reported as isolated and passive, they exhibit deprivation and withdrawal, next to a very low behavioral repertoire, emphasizing few opportunities of positive interactions with the surrounding environment. Thus, their clinical conditions may highly hamper their social image, desirability, and status [6-7-8].

The objective of this chapter is to investigate some issues related to the FXS. Specifically, the following features related to FXS will be addressed and critically discussed: (a) molecular and genetic features, (b) brain structure, (c) intellectual development, (d) social communication, (e) challenging behavior, (f) pharmacological intervention and (g) cognitive-behavioral intervention.

2. MOLECULAR AND GENETIC FEATURES

FXS is the most frequent cause of sex-linked intellectual disabilities. In the majority of the cases, the mutation responsible for the Martin Bell syndrome is produced when an expansion of the (CGG)n repetition is present in the region 5' of the exón 1 of the gene for X-fragile mental retardation 1 (FMR1), together with a hypermethylation in the CpG promoter region of the gene. The result of this situation is the absence of FMRP protein coded by the gene. The correlation between length of the (CGG)n sequences and of the X-fragile phenotype has permitted a more specific diagnosis of affected and carrier individuals by means of direct DNA analysis. Nevertheless, the molecular genetic basis of the instability and expansion of the (CGG)n sequence represents a problem not resolved yet. Two polymorphic microsatellite (AC)n repetitions, FRAXAC1 and

FRAXAC2 that flank the FMR-1 gene have been recently described. It has been suggested that some haplotypes of FRAXAC1 and FRAXAC2 could be associated to long (CGG)n repetitions and these haplotypes would confer more instability to the repeated fragment, thus increasing the probability of expansion. It has also been described that the (CGG)n repetition of the FMR-1 gene is interrupted by AGG trinucleotides and that the loss of one AGG would be an important mutational event in the generation of predisposing unstable alleles of the X-fragile syndrome [9].

3. BRAIN STRUCTURE

Brain imaging studies establish an unambiguous link between FXS and abnormalities of brain morphology. In the context of overall normal brain size in individuals with FXS, disproportionate volume increases are observed in the caudate nucleus, whereas decreases are recorded in the superior temporal gyrus, amygdala, and cerebellar vermis. These neuroanatomic variations in FXS are robust, particularly those observed in the caudate, and can be linked to variation in measures of FMR1 expression, age, cognition, and behavior. Further, results from diffusion tensor imaging show a reduced fractional anisotropy within pre-frontal caudate and parietal pathways in FXS. Abnormalities in white matter connectivity, putatively related to FMRP's function in regulating axonal pathfinding may further disrupt the integrity of critical neurofunctional networks involved in executive function and visuospatial processing in FXS [10].

Identifiable associations among measures of FMRP, neuroanatomy, cognition, and behavior in FXS suggest that the morphologic findings described above are clinically meaningful. Thus, an increasing degree of aberrant brain morphology is associated with lower IQ and FMRP and higher levels of behavioral dysfunction. In contrast, larger caudate size is associated with higher IQ for controls [11]. Data suggest that increases in caudate volume in individuals with FXS reflect aberrant neuronal organization. Despite the high prevalence of FXS as a heritable genetic disorder, detailed postmortem studies of humans are rare [12].

4. Intellectual Development

Individuals with FXS may present a continuum from learning disabilities in the context of a normal intelligence quotient (IQ) to severe intellectual disability, with an average IQ of 40 in males who have complete silencing of the FMR1 gene. Females, who tend to be less affected, generally have an IQ which is normal or borderline with learning difficulties. The main difficulties in individuals with FXS are with working and short-term memory, executive functions, visual memory, visual-spatial relationships, and mathematics, with verbal abilities being relatively unaffected.

Data on intellectual development in FXS are limited. However, there is some evidence that standardized IQ decreases over the time in a large part of the cases, apparently as a result of slowed intellectual development. A longitudinal study looking at pairs of siblings, where one child was affected and the other was not, found that affected children had an intellectual learning rate which was 55% slower than unaffected children [13-14]. Individuals with FXS often demonstrated language and communicative problems. This may be related to muscle function of the mouth and frontal-lobe deficits [15].

5. Social Communication

The early social communication may be an early indicator of ASD in infants with FXS. In children and adults with FXS, social communication (i.e., pragmatics) is impaired, and these impairments are greater for individuals with co- morbid ASD [16-17]. However, the early social communication profile of infants and young children with FXS is largely unknown with few studies examining social communication at this age period [18-19-20]. Marschik et al., [19] investigated children with FXS 12 months or younger and found that most communication consisted of prelinguistic vocalizations with restricted gesture use. In slightly older children (21–77 months), deficits in reciprocity and gestures have also been reported. Within gesture use, it appears that children with FXS (15–41 months) use more contact gestures (i.e., giving, pushing away, touching an adult hand) and have to transition to more advanced gestures (i.e., representational gestures and distal pointing) yet. Interestingly, using eye gaze shifts, eye gaze to a person's face that alternates between the person and an object or the purposes of behavior requests, joint attention, and responding to communication have been reported as relatively intact in infants and young children with FXS [19-20]. These findings are opposite to data on older children, adolescents, and adults who evidenced difficulties using eye gaze for initiating and maintaining social interactions [21-22]. Furthermore, gaze avoidance as core of the FXS phenotype was outlined. However, these studies have primarily focused on eye gaze in FXS outside of a communication context. Further investigations in infants during social communication are warranted [23-24].

6. Challenging Behavior

FXS is the most common inherited cause of intellectual disability [25] and a genetic condition in which challenging behaviors are frequently reported [26]. The condition is caused by a CGG triplet expansion on the FMR1 gene, located on the long arm of the X chromosome. As a result of this expansion, the gene typically becomes methylated, resulting in cessation or suppression of its protein product FMRP, which is important in many aspects of development and brain function [27-28]. As a result of the X-linked nature of the condition, females show more unclear and variable effects. The widespread effects of the genetic mutation are associated with a phenotype including varying degrees of intellectual disability, anxiety, attention deficits and autistic-like behavior [29-30].

Self-injurious behavior (SIB), aggression and destructive behavior have been described in individuals with this condition [26]. Indeed, hand-biting has been described as part of the behavioral phenotype [31]. It is reported by clinicians and parents that SIB and aggressive outbursts in FXS are often associated with sensory stimulation or unexpected change, which leads to the individual feeling overwhelmed and, in turn, hyper-aroused [32] and stressed [26]. Data suggested that changes to the physiology of the stress response may be associated with the operant conditioning of challenging behaviors with an escape function, within this group [33-34-35]. Additionally, a number of characteristics commonly associated with FXS have been identified as risk factors for engagement in challenging behavior, among people with intellectual disabilities [36]. These features include: (a) autism [37], and (b) over-activity and impulsivity [38]. The heightened presence of these risk factors in FXS, as well as the syndrome-specific factors discussed, evidence several possible associations between FXS and challenging behaviors [39].

Self-injurious and aggressive behaviors are commonly observed in FXS. However, little is known about the persistence of these behaviors and associated risk markers. Hayley et al., [40] established the prevalence and persistence of self-injurious and aggressive behaviors over eight years in males with FXS, and associations with risk markers. Results showed 77% and 69% persistence rates for self-injurious and aggressive behavior, respectively. Baseline levels of repetitive behavior predicted persistent self-injurious behavior. Chronological age, impulsivity and overactivity were associated with persistent aggressive behavior but only impulsivity predicted persistence. This is the first study to document the persistence of self-injurious and aggressive behavior in FXS over the medium to long term and to identify behavioral risk markers that might facilitate targeted early intervention.

7. Pharmacological Interventions

The pharmacological treatments investigated to date which targeted symptoms of FXS are extremely limited. Although mild reduction of symptoms can be recorded in individuals with FXS who are treated with antidepressants or stimulants, there is a pressing need for new, more effective, disease-specific treatments in young children with this condition [12]. Medical research (e.g., Hagerman et al., 2009) indicates that to date the most effective drug therapies include antagonist molecules of glutamate receptors used to reduce aggressive and repetitive behaviors, mood stabilizers such as lithium, drugs that inhibit the reuptake of serotonin to control anxiety and depressive states. Consultation with a specialized neurologist is considered crucial in order to identify the most appropriate drug therapy [41].

8. Cognitive-Behavioral Interventions

The cognitive-behavioral interventions are effective for children with FXS. Cognitive-Behavioral Therapy (CBT) constitutes a large and heterogeneous corpus of theoretical approaches combined by assumptions resulting from psychological research carried out in the cognitive field. In this process of integration between theoretical and practical knowledge, CBT orientations are characterized by a core of fundamental assumptions. The first assumption postulates that cognitive activity affects behavior; the second states that cognitive activity can be both controlled and modified; the third assumption argues that it is possible to obtain the desired behavioral changes through a cognitive modification [42].

A large body of literature has emerged documenting the influence of environmental factors on behavior disorders shown by individuals with developmental disabilities [43-44]. These studies showed that many behavior disorders (e.g., aggression, self-injury, and stereotypic behaviors) are influenced by antecedent and consequent social-environmental events.

These environmental events include antecedent task or social demands, contingent removal of task or social demands, low levels of antecedent attention, concomitant presentation of attention, changes in routines, and low levels of sensory stimulation. Manipulation of these environmental events can dramatically reduce the occurrence of these challenging behaviors [45-46].

For example, Hessl et al., [47] found that challenging behaviors in boys with FXS were consistently associated with environmental factors (education/therapeutic services and maternal psychological problems) rather than biological factors (FMRP). Additionally, children with FXS showed higher rates of challenging behavior during social demand situations than non-social situations [48], demonstrating that their behavior is responsive to changes in the social environment. Furthermore, across two studies that conducted functional analyses of challenging behavior in children with FXS, the majority of children with FXS exhibited challenging behavior that functioned to escape demands or access tangible items, with fewer showing social-escape behavior or attention-maintained challenging behavior. Although biological factors play a role in FXS, these studies demonstrate that the behavior of individuals with FXS can also be influenced by the environment and often serves an operant function. This suggests that the behavior of individuals with FXS can be altered using behavioral interventions [49].

CONCLUSION AND DISCUSSION

Fragile X Syndrome is a hereditary genetic condition, that is, it is transmitted from parents to children, and is the cause of cognitive disabilities, learning and relationship problems. The current chapter included information concerning the Fragile X Syndrome within seven basic macro-areas: (1) Molecular and Genetic Features, (2) Brain Structure, (3) Intellectual Development, (4) Social Communication, (5) Challenging Behavior, (6) Pharmacological Interventions, and (7)

Cognitive-Behavioral Interventions. These areas developed within the chapter have provided important insights into the Fragile X Syndrome.

First, Fragile X Syndrome is considered the leading hereditary cause, resulting from a single gene, of intellectual disability and some forms of autism. It is determined by the silencing of the FMR1 gene located on the long arm of the X chromosome (q27.3), which encodes the FMRP protein, which in turn has the function of controlling the translation of specific messengers (Salcedo-Arellano et al., 2019). More specifically, FXS would be due to the expansion of the trinucleotide CGG (cytosine-guanine-guanine) in the untranslated portion 5 of this gene, which tends to change in amplitude in the passage from one generation to another [50].

Second, as for the neuroanatomical part of the disease, disproportionate increases in volume are observed in the caudate nucleus, while decreases are recorded in the superior temporal gyrus, amygdala and cerebellar worm [11]. Third, on the psychological-cognitive axis, it was instead observed that: approximately 60% of individuals with XFS have a concomitant diagnosis of autism while 70% manifest a comorbidity with ADHD. Concomitant psychiatric disorders such as anxiety, depression, and obsessive-compulsive disorder may be found. Moreover, 85% of males and 30% of females have medium-severe intellectual disability, while 25% of females the IQ is within the normal range [51].

Fourth, there are difficulties in learning, in the ability to process information, in communication and language development. Verbal skills are higher than visuospatial skills, despite the fact that the language of people with FXS presents itself as repetitive, tangential and persevering [52].

Fifth, on the behavioral level, the presence of repetitive and stereotyped behaviors, difficulty in changing the routine, poor eye contact, symptoms shared with autism spectrum disorders were acknowledged. Sixth, as regards the possibility of pharmacological treatment, to date, there is no cure for FXS and its treatment is aimed at improving the symptoms associated with it [53].

Seventh, cognitive-behavioral therapy helps the patient to identify their dysfunctional thoughts and replace them with more adaptive thought processes. The goal is to carry out a real cognitive restructuring that modifies not only the mental states, but also the emotional and behavioral components. However, it can only be used with individuals with an adequate cognitive level [52].

REFERENCES

[1] Moskowitz L J, Jones E A. Uncovering the evidence for behavioral interventions with individuals with fragile X syndrome: a systematic review. *Research in Developmental Disabilities*. 2015: 38: 223– 241.

[2] Oakes A, Ma M, McDuffie A, MacHalicek W, Abbeduto L. Providing a parent implemented language intervention to a young male with fragile X syndrome: brief report. *Developmental Neurorehabilitation*. 2015:18: 65–68.

[3] Hagerman R J, Polussa J. Treatment of the psychiatric problems associated with fragile X syndrome. *Current Opinion in Psychiatry*. 2015: 28: 107–112

[4] Cornish, K. M., Turk, J., Wilding, J., Sudhalter, V., Munir, F., Kooy, F., & Hagerman, R. (2004).

[5] Haessler F, Gaese F, Huss M, Kretschmar C, Brinkman M, Peters H, Pittrow D. Characterization, treatment patterns, and patient-related outcomes of patients with fragile X syndrome in Germany: Final results of the observational EXPLAIN-FXS study. *BMC Psychiatry*. 2016: 16(1): 12-24.

[6] Frielink N, Embregts P. Modification of motivational interviewing for use with people with mild intellectual disability and challenging behavior. *Journal of Intellectual and Developmental Disability*. 2013: 38: 279–291.

[7] Lancioni G E, O'Reilly M F, Singh N N, Sigafoos J, Buonocunto F, Sacco V, et al. Technology-aided leisure and communication opportunities for two post-coma persons emerged from a minimally

conscious state and affected by multiple disabilities. *Research in Developmental Disabilities.* 2013: 34: 809–816.

[8] Stasolla F, Perilli V, Damiani R, Caffò A O, Di Leone A, Albano V, et al. A microswitch-cluster program to enhance object manipulation and to reduce hand mouthing by three boys with autism spectrum disorders and intellectual disabilities. *Research in Autism Spectrum Disorders.* 2014: 8: 1071–1078.

[9] Jara L, Avendano I B, Aspillaga M H, Blanco R. *Molecular and genetic features of fragile X syndrome*: a review. Revista medica de Chile. 1996: 124(7): 865-72).

[10] Brown V, Jin P, Ceman S, et al. Microarray identification of FMRP-associated brain mRNAs and altered mRNA translational profiles in fragile X syndrome. *Cell.* 2001: 107(4): 477–87.

[11] Reiss A L, Abrams M T, Greenlaw R, et al. Neurodevelopmental effects of the FMR-1 full mutation in humans. *National Medicine.* 1995: 1(2): 159–67.

[12] Allan L, Reiss M D, Scott S, Hall P. *Fragile X Syndrome: Assessment and Treatment Implications.* Child and Adolescent Psychiatric Clinics of North America. 2007: 16: 663-75.

[13] Garber K B, Visootsak J, Warren S T (June 2008). "Fragile X syndrome". *European Journal of Human Genetics.* 16 (6): 666–72.

[14] Hall S S, Burns D D, Lightbody A A, Reiss A L. Longitudinal changes in intellectual development in children with Fragile X syndrome. *Journal of Abnormal Child Psychology.* 2008: 36(6): 927–39.

[15] Abbeduto L, Hagerman R J. Language and communication in fragile X syndrome. *Mental Retardation and Developmental Disabilities Research Reviews.* 1997: 3(4): 313–322.

[16] Klusek J, Martin G E, Losh M. A comparison of pragmatic language in boys with autism and fragile X syndrome. *Jounral of Speech, Language, and Hearing Research*, 2014: 57(3): 1692–1707.

[17] Martin G E, Losh M, Estigarribia B, Sideris J, Roberts J. Longitudinal profiles of expressive vocabulary, syntax and pragmatic language in boys with fragile X syndrome or Down

syndrome. *International Journal of Language & Communication Disorders.* 2013: 48(4): 432–443.

[18] Lenthrope J L, Brady N C. Relationships between early gestures and later language in children with fragile X syndrome. *American Journal of Speech- Language Pathology.* 2010: 19(2): 135–142.

[19] Marschik P B, Bartl-Pokorny K D, Sigafoos J, Urlesberger L, Pokorny F, Didden R. Development of socio-communicative skills in 9- to 12-month- old individuals with fragile X syndrome. *Research in Developmental Disabilities.* 2014: 35(3): 597–602.

[20] Roberts J E, Mirrett P, Anderson K, Burchinal M, Neebe E. Early communication, symbolic behavior, and social profiles of young males with fragile X syndrome. *American Journal of Speech- Language Pathology.* 2002: 11(3): 295–304.

[21] Hall S S, Frank M C, Pusiol G T, Farzin F, Lightbody A A, Reiss A L. Quantifying naturalistic social gaze in fragile X syndrome using a novel eye tracking paradigm. *American Journal of Medical Genetic.* 2015: 168(7): 564–572.

[22] Williams T A, Porter M A, Langdon R. Viewing social scenes: A visual scan-path study comparing fragile X syndrome and Williams syndrome. *Journal of Autism and Developmental Disorders.* 2013: 43(8): 1880–1894.

[23] Cohen I, Fisch G, Sudhalter V, Wolf-Scein EG, Hanson D, Hagerman R. Social gaze, social avoidance, and repetitive behaviors in fragile X males: A controlled study. *American Journal on Mental Retardation.* 1988: 92(5): 436–446.

[24] Murphy M, Abbeduto L, Schroeder S, Serlin R. Contribution of social and information-processing factors to eye-gaze avoidance in fragile X syndrome. *American Journal on Mental Retardation.* 2007: 112(5): 349–360.

[25] Mazzocco M M. Advances in research on fragile X syndrome. *Mental Retardation and Developmental Disability Research.* 2000: 6: 96–106.

[26] Hessl D, Dyer-Friedman J, Glaser B, Wisbeck J, Barajas R G, Taylor A. The influence of environmental and genetic factors on behavior

problems and autistic symptoms in boys and girls with fragile X syndrome. *Pediatrics.* 2001: 108(5): 88.

[27] Santoro M R, Bray S. M., & Warren, S. T. Molecular mechanisms of Fragile X Syndrome: A twenty-year perspective. *Annual Review of Pathology: Mechanisms of Disease.* 2012: 7: 219–245.

[28] Verkerk A J, Pieretti M, Sutcliffe J S, Fu Y H, Kuhl D P, Pizzuti A. Identification of a gene (FMR-1) containing a CGG repeat coincident with a breakpoint cluster region exhibiting length variation in fragile X syndrome. *Cell.* 1991: 65: 905–914.

[29] Bailey D B, Raspa M, Bishop E M D, Martin S, Wheeler A, Sacco P. Health and economic consequences of fragile X syndrome for caregivers. *Journal of Developmental & Behavioral Pediatrics.* 2012: 33(9): 705–712.

[30] Cordeiro L, Ballinger E, Hagerman R, Hessl D. Clinical assessment of DSM-IV anxiety disorders in fragile X syndrome: Prevalence and characterization. *Journal of Neurodevelopmental Disorders.* 2010: 3(1): 57.

[31] Hagerman R J. *Fragile X syndrome: Diagnosis, treatment, and research* (pp.1–109). Baltimore: JHU Press. 2002.

[32] Miller L J, McIntosh D N, McGrath J, Shyu V, Lampe M, Taylor AK. Electrodermal responses to sensory stimuli in individuals with fragile X syndrome. *American Journal of Medical Genetics.* 1999: 83: 268–279.

[33] Hardiman R L, McGill P. The topographies and operant functions of challenging behaviours in fragile X syndrome: A systematic review and analysis of existing data. *Journal of Intellectual & Developmental Disability.* 2017: 42(2): 190–203.

[34] Langthorne P, McGill P. An indirect examination of the function of problem behavior associated with fragile X syndrome and Smith-Magenis syndrome. *Journal of Autism and Developmental Disorders.* 2012: 42(2): 201–209.

[35] Langthorne P, McGill P, O'Reilly M F, Lang R, Machalicek W, Chan J M, Rispoli M. Examining the function of problem behavior in fragile X syndrome: Preliminary experimental analysis. *American Journal of Intellectual and Developmental Disabilities.* 2011: 116(1): 65–80.

[36] McClintock K, Hall S, & Oliver C. Risk markers associated with challenging behaviors in people with intellectual disabilities: A meta-analytic study. *Journal of Intellectual Disability Research.* 2003: 47(6): 405–416.

[37] Oliver C, Berg K, Moss J, Arron K, Burbidge C. Delineation of behavioral phenotypes in genetic syndromes: Characteristics of autism spectrum disorder, affect and hyperactivity. *Journal of Autism and Developmental Disorders.* 2011: 41(8): 1019–1032.

[38] Baumgardner T L, Reiss A L, Freund L S. Specification of the neurobehavioral phenotype in males with fragile X syndrome. *Pediatrics.* 1995: 5: 744–752.

[39] Hardiman R L, McGrill P. How common are challenging behaviors amongst individuals with Fragile X Syndrome? A systematic review. *Research in Developmental Disabilities.* 2018: 76: 99-109.

[40] Hayley C, Karakatsani E, Singla G, Oliver C. The Persistence of Self-injurious and Aggressive Behavior in Males with Fragile X Syndrome Over 8 Years: A Longitudinal Study of Prevalence and Predictive Risk Markers. *Journal of Autism and Developmental Disorders.* 2019: 49: 2913-2922.

[41] *Hagerman R J, Berry-Kravis E, Kaufmann W E, Ono M Y, Tartaglia N, Lachiewicz A, Picker J. Advances in the treatment of fragile X syndrome. Pediatrics. 2009: 123(1): 378-390.*

[42] Villa V, Caretti A. Gli interventi psicologici: il paradigma cognitivo-comportamentale. *Clinica psicologica dell'obesità.* Springer-Verlag. 2012: 105-119.

[43] Carr E G, Durand V M. The social-communicative basis of severe behavior problems in children. In: Reiss S, Bootzin R, editors. *Theoretical issues in behavior therapy.* New York: Academic Press. 1985.

[44] Hanley GP, Iwata BA, McCord BE. Functional analysis of problem behavior: a review. *J. Appl. Behav. Anal.* 2003: 36: 147–85.

[45] Taylor JC, Carr EG. Severe problem behaviors related to social interaction: I. Attention seeking and social avoidance. *Behav. Modif.* 1992: 16: 305–35.

[46] Call N A, Wacker DP, Ringdahl JE, et al. An assessment of antecedent events influencing noncompliance in an outpatient clinic. *J. Appl. Behav. Anal.* 2004: 37: 145–58.

[47] Hall S S, Oliver C, Murphy G. Early development of self-injurious behavior: An empirical study. *American Journal on Mental Retardation.* 2001: 106(2): 189– 199.

[48] Hall S S, DeBernardis G M, Reiss A L. The acquisition of stimulus equivalence in individuals with fragile X syndrome. *Journal of Intellectual Disability Research.* 2006: 50(9): 643–651.

[49] Langthorne P, McGill P. An indirect examination of the function of problem behavior associated with fragile X syndrome and Smith–Magenis syndrome. *Journal of Autism and Developmental Disorders.* 2012: 42: 201–209.

[50] Nolin S L. Expansion of the Fragile X CGG Repeat in Females with Premutation or Intermediate Alleles. *Am. J. Hum. Genet.* 2003: 72: 454-464.

[51] Bailey J, Raspa M, Olmsted M, Holiday D B. Co-occurring conditions associated with FMR1 gene variations: findings from a national parent survey. *American journal of medical genetics part A.* 2008: 146(16): 2060-2069.

[52] Abbeduto L, McDuffie A, Thurman AJ, Kover ST. Language development in individuals with intellectual and developmental disabilities: From phenotypes to treatments. In *International review of research in developmental disabilities* (Vol. 50, pp. 71-118). Academic Press. 2016.

[53] Corona F, De Giuseppe T. L'identikit dell'X Fragile tra comprensione genetica, potenzialità fenotipiche, bisogni potenziali ed emergenze educative inclusivo-socio-emotive. *Italian Journal of Special Education For Inclusion*, 2018: 6(1): 51-62. [The identikit of Fragile X between genetic understanding, phenotypic potential, potential needs and inclusive-socio-emotional educational emergencies]

In: Fragile X Syndrome
Editor: Fabrizio Stasolla

ISBN: 978-1-68507-572-9
© 2022 Nova Science Publishers, Inc.

Chapter 5

MICROSWITCH-CLUSTER TECHNOLOGY TO PROMOTE CONSTRUCTIVE ENGAGEMENT AND REDUCE MOUTHING IN TWO CHILDREN WITH FRAGILE X SYNDROME AND DEVELOPMENTAL DISABILITIES

Donatella Ciarmoli[*] *and Fabrizio Stasolla*
"Giustino Fortunato" University of Benvento, Italy

ABSTRACT

Background

Fragile X syndrome (FXS) is a rare genetic disease and represents one of the frequent causes of severe to profound developmental disabilities. Hyperactivity, impulsivity, and anxiety are included,

---

[*] Corresponding Author's E-mail: d.ciarmoli1@studenti.unifortunato.eu.

Assistive technology (AT) can reduce the effect of negative outcomes and provides improved quality of life.

Objectives

To extend the use of AT for promoting a new adaptive response and to reduce hand mouthing by two boys with fragile X syndrome and severe to profound developmental disabilities.

Method

A microswitch-cluster technology was implemented to (a) promote an adaptive responding, (b) reduce challenging behaviors, and (c) evaluate the effects of the intervention on positive participation as an outcome measure of the quality of life in two children with fragile X syndrome. The study was conducted according to a non-concurrent multiple baseline design across participants followed by intervention and cross-over phases, where the associations between behavioral responses and environmental consequences were systematically inverted.

Results

Data evidenced an improved adaptive responding and a decreased challenging behavior in both participants, who enhanced their positive participation.

Conclusion

A microswitch-cluster technology was effective and suitable to increase an adaptive responding and reduce a challenging behavior in participants diagnosed with fragile X.

1. INTRODUCTION

Fragile X syndrome (FXS) is a genetic disorder. It is caused by an excessive length of a repetitive sequence of trinucleotides (CGG) in a specific gene (FMR1), matched to FMR1 protein, which is primarily responsible for the regular brain developing and functioning. It represents one of the most frequent causes of developmental disabilities with learning difficulties, and may have consequences on intellectual, communicative and social functioning. Additionally, anxiety, hyperactivity, seizures, gaze avoidance and autism spectrum disorders are commonly described within its patterns, basically occurring in males. FXS physical characteristics usually include long and narrow visage, large ears, prominent jaws and foreheads. Stereotypic behaviors, aggression and self-injuries are equally described among this population [1-3]. Accordingly, individuals with FXS may be fully considered as affected by severe to profound developmental disabilities [4]. Thus, individuals with FXS may be acknowledged within the range of multiple disabilities. Children with multiple disabilities may present a certain number of challenges to rehabilitation staff [5]. For example, they can exhibit lack of positive interaction with surrounding objects, stereotyped behaviors, and passivity. A critical rehabilitative goal is to point out an effective strategy that may help those individuals to acquire constructive engagement with environmental stimulation, such as object manipulation. Positive stimulation (i.e., environmental events enabling and motivating the performance by increasing and consolidating behavioral responses over the time) [6].

To emphasize such perspective, one may envisage the use of assistive technology-based interventions (AT), aimed at monitoring the aforementioned behaviors and consequently providing the contingent stimulation, based on learning principles [7]. AT generally includes any piece, device, equipment or tool capable of enabling positive participation, favorable occupation, and constructive engagement in individuals with multiple disabilities [8]. Microswitches represent basic forms of AT enabling persons with severe to profound developmental and/or multiple disabilities to positively interact with external environment. For example, brief periods of positive stimulation (e.g., 7–10 s) may be automatically delivered by an electronic system contingently on small behavioral responses (e.g., eye blinking, hand closing) detected by specific tools (e.g., optic or pressure sensors) [9-10]. In other words, a participant with severe to profound intellectual disabilities will be capable to determine the provision of positive environmental events independently [11-12]. Within this framework, microswitch-cluster technology (MCT) pursues the dual simultaneous goal of promoting an adaptive response and reducing a challenging behavior [7].

For example, Perrilli et al. [13] further extended the use of microswitch-cluster technology for promoting occupational activities and reducing hand biting in six adolescents with fragile X syndrome and severe to profound developmental disabilities. The primary rehabilitative goal was to enhance the adaptive response (i.e., inserting three different objects in the three containers within a 4 s time interval). The secondary objective was to evaluate the effects of the intervention on indices of positive participation as an outcome measure of the participants 'quality of life. Finally, a social validation assessment involving sixty-six external raters was conducted. The study was carried out according to an ABB^1AB^1 experimental sequence for each participant. Thus, A indicated baselines, B indicated the intervention focused on promoting the adaptive response irrespective of the challenging behavior, and B^1 indicated the cluster phases with the provision of positive stimulation only if the adaptive response was exhibited free of the challenging behavior. A one-year follow-up was implemented. Results showed an improved performance for all the participants, which was maintained over the time. Indices of positive participation increased as well. Social raters favorably scored the use of the microswitch-cluster technology.

Stasolla, Perilli, Damiani, and Albano [14], exposed three participants with FXS (aged of 8.8, 9.4 and 10.5 respectively) to an AT-based rehabilitative strategy for promoting a new adaptive response (i.e., inserting two different objects in two different containers within a 3 s time interval). A three-month follow-up and a social validation assessment involving 30 parents of children with severe to profound developmental disabilities were additionally conducted. Data showed that all participants increased the adaptive responding and reduced the stereotypic behaviors during the intervention phases. They all consolidated their performance within the follow-up and social raters favorably scored the use of AT. The aforementioned empirical evidences suggest that further extensions of the AT for children with FXS is undoubtedly warranted. Recently, Stasolla et al. [15] positively extended the implementation of an MBP to three new participants with FXS for (a) promoting a new adaptive response (i.e., insert two different objects in two containers available, within 3 s), (b) monitoring its effect on participants' positive mood, (c) conducting a three-month follow-up, and (d) assessing a social validation procedure involving 30 parents of children with developmental disabilities as external raters. All the participants profitably learned the use of the technology for occupational purposes and consolidated it during the follow-up. The MBP had beneficial consequences on participants' mood. Social raters favorably endorsed the use of the MBP. Despite the aforementioned encouraging and promising findings, new extensions were recommended.

In light of the above, this study implemented a rehabilitation intervention based on the use of MCT in two children with fragile X syndrome, and was aimed at pursuing the following objectives: (a) to promote an adaptive responding for both participants, that is, the manipulation of objects; (b) to decrease stereotyped behaviors exhibited by the participants involved (i.e., mouthing); and (c) to monitor the intervention's effects on the participant's indices of happiness.

2. METHOD

2.1. Participants and Setting

The eligibility criteria assessed at the beginning of the study were (a) a diagnosis of FXS, (b) a chronological age comprised between 6 and 13 years old (i.e., the study was focused on children with FXS), (c) severe to profound intellectual and developmental disabilities, (d) hand-biting stereotypic behavior reported by parents and caregivers, and (e) the capacity of managing familiar objects if adequately rewarded (i.e., the capacity of keeping up a familiar object if rewarded) (i.e., being highly motivated), without the caregivers' assistance. Accordingly, two children

(Adam and Brian) who were aged 8,5 and 9,6 at the beginning of the study were recruited. Both were diagnosed with FXS full mutation based on DNA results and laboratory tests. Additionally, they were mosaic since they presented a full mutation and a premutation, consistent with the documented prevalence among males available in the literature. Although no IQ score was available because no test was feasible, due to their clinical conditions, the Vineland Adaptive Behavior Scale (VABS) revealed a mental age of 1.3 (Adam), and 1.5 (Brian). Accordingly, they were estimated within the severe to profound range of developmental and intellectual disabilities.

They presented lack of speech, communication inabilities, unawareness of sphincter control, failure of independent ambulation. Both exhibited hand and objects mouthing as a related stereotypic behavior and attended regular classes with a special educational program supervised by a support teacher 24 h per week. Adam was exposed to speech sessions twice a week, Brian followed a physiotherapy program once per week. Both were described by their parents and caregivers as quite isolated and passive. They were reported to the research team by their neurologist and their psychologist. Both lived in their homes with their parents who were enthusiastic of the proposed technology-aided cluster program. In fact, they signed a formal consent for the participation of their children to the rehabilitative intervention, which was approved by a local scientific and ethic committee and was carried out according to Helsinki Declaration and its later amendments [16-17].

2.2. Selection of Stimuli

An informal parents' interview preceded a formal preference screening [18]. Thus, within a 10 min session 30–40 non-consecutive presentations of preferred stimuli occurred, with 15–20 s rest interval across each presentation. Stimuli were retained whether they caused participants' alerting, orientation and/or smiling reactions, at least in the 70% of their presentations. For both participants, music, videos, and colored lights by the children were selected.

2.3. Technology and Response

In this intervention, for both participants (a) the adaptive response consisted of objects' manipulation; (b) the challenging behavior consisted of hands and objects' mouthing. The technology consisted of three objects (a puppet, a ball, and a pen) each of which was associated with a pleasant stimulus (music, video, or colored lights), activable through a wobble (i.e., a pressure) microswitch, an optic sensor fixed on the corner of the participant's lip, a laptop, visible but inaccessible to the participants, and an interface that connected the microswitches to the laptop. The laptop was equipped with a 17-inch monitor and a Clicker 5 software package (Crick House, Moulton Park, Northampton, UK). Both pressure and optic microswitches constituted the cluster technology.

The rationale for choosing the adaptive response was (a) preventing passivity, (b) promoting occupational activities, (c) improving constructive engagement, and (d) teaching a functional task [19].

2.4. Experimental Conditions

The study, which lasted approximately 5 months, was carried out according to a non-concurrent multiple baseline design across participants with baseline phases longer for Bernard with respect to those occurred for Adam [20]. Thus, each baseline phase for Adam included 5 sessions, while the Bernard ones included 8 sessions. The program introduced an initial intervention phase, in which the responses of the participants led to different environmental consequences. Once the responses were consolidated a cross over phase occurred. Thus, a systematic inversion between behavioral response and environmental consequences occurred. Subsequently, a new baseline phase for both participants was conducted, with a different length between participants. Following the new baseline, a new intervention phase was carried out, with a new cross over phase. Overall, 82 sessions were collected for Adam and 90 sessions for Bernard, depending on the different length of both baseline phases for each participant.

2.4.1. First Baseline

During the baseline, the technology was available (i.e., objects with wobble and optic sensors), but the behavioral responses eventually exhibited by both participants did not have any environmental consequences. Baseline phase for Adam included 5 sessions, while baseline phase for Bernard included 8 sessions. Data recording included (a) the number of manipulated objects, (b) the percentages of intervals with stereotypic behaviors, and (c) the percentages of intervals with indices of happiness (see above Section 2.3).

2.4.2. First Intervention

During the first phase of intervention, the conditions were identical to the baseline, except for the environmental consequences. That is, if Adam and/or Bernard manipulated the puppet, they received 10s of video, if they manipulated the ball they would receive 10s of favorite music stimulation, and if they manipulated the pen they would receive 10s of colored light stimulation. This phase included 21 sessions for each participant.

2.4.3. First Cross Over

During the first crossover phase, the experimental conditions were identical to those of the first intervention, except for the association between behavioral responses and environmental consequences. That is, by manipulating the puppet, Adam and Bernard received a stimulation period of 10 seconds of music. If the ball was managed, they received 10 s of stimulation of colored lights. Finally, if they managed the pen they received 10s of stimulation of favorite videos. This phase included 30 sessions for each participant.

2.4.4. Second Baseline

At the end of the crossover phase, a new baseline was made for both participants. The experimental conditions were identical to those of the first baseline, as well as its length for each participant. That is, the new baseline for Adam included 5 sessions, while the new baseline for Bernard included 8 sessions.

2.4.5. Second Cross Over

During the second cross over, experimental conditions were identical to those of the first cross over (see above Section 2.4.3). Thus, by manipulating the puppet, Adam and Bernard received a stimulation period of 10 seconds of music. If the ball was manipulated. They received 10 s of stimulation with the colored lights. Lastly, if they manipulated the pen, they received 10s of stimulation of favorite videos. This phase included 30 sessions for each participant.

3. RESULTS

Data were summarized over blocks of sessions and plotted in Figures 1, 2, 3, and 4. Mean scores and ranges of the participants' performances (i.e., adaptive responding, challenging behavior, and indices of positive participation) were included in Tables 1, 2 and 3. For both participants (Adam and Brian), the data showed an increased adaptive responding during the intervention and cluster phases, compared to baselines. Challenging behavior was drastically reduced. Positive participation increased significantly. The differences between the baselines on the one hand and the intervention and cluster phases on the other were statistically significant ($p < .01$) for the Kolmogorov-Smirnov test (Siegel and Castellan 1988).

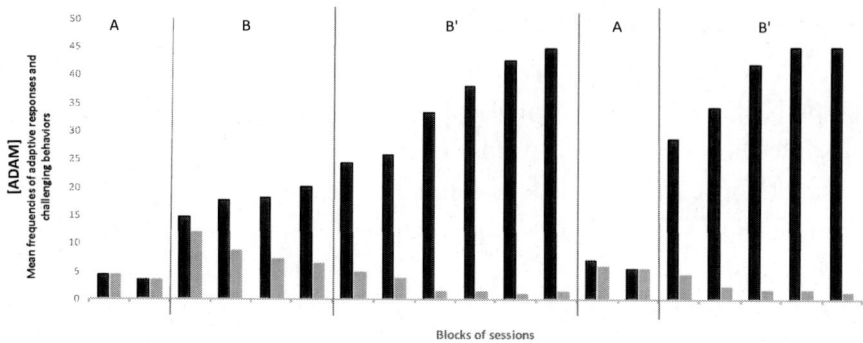

Figure 1. The graph summarizes the data about performance for Adam. The black and the light bars indicate the mean frequencies of adaptive responses and challenging behavior, respectively, over blocks of sessions for the two baselines phase and the three intervention phases.

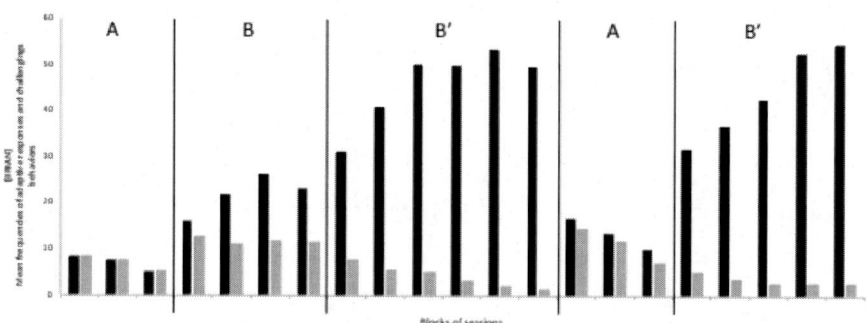

Figure 2. The graph summarizes the data about performance for Brian. The black and the light bars indicate the mean frequencies of adaptive responses and challenging behavior, respectively, over blocks of sessions for the two baselines phase and the three intervention phases.

Microswitch-Cluster Technology to Promote ... 121

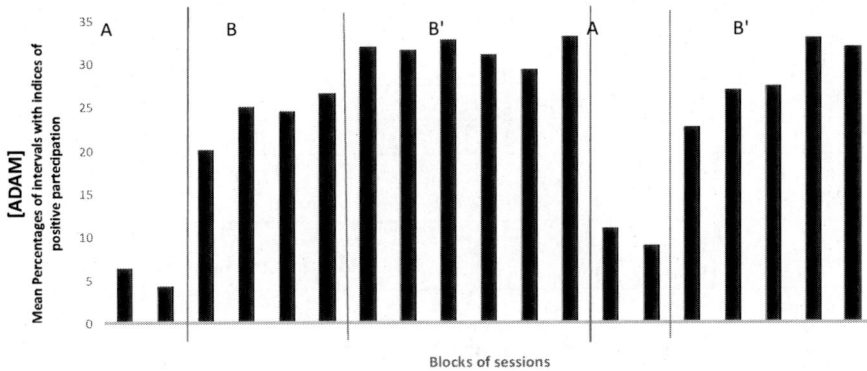

Figure 3. The graph summarizes the data about the participation for Adam. The black diamonds refer to the mean percentage of intervals with indices of positive participation over blocks of sessions for the two baseline phases and the three intervention phases.

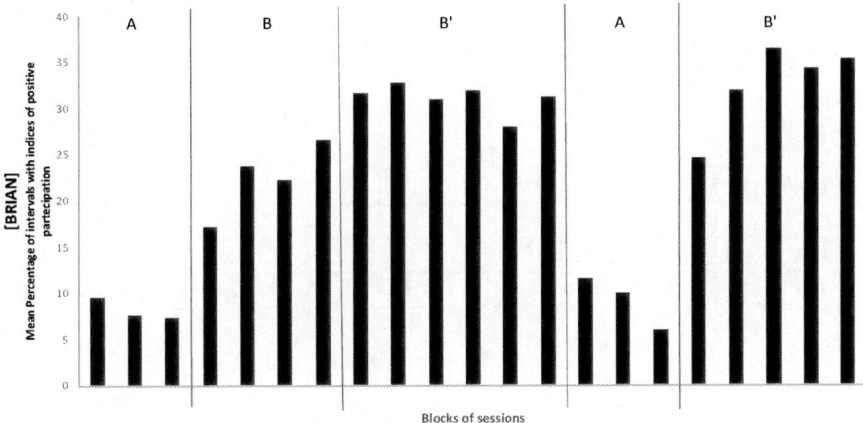

Figure 1. The graph summarizes the data about the participation for Brian the black diamonds refer to the mean percentage of intervals with indices of positive participation over blocks of sessions for the two baseline phases and the three intervention phases.

Table 1. Mean values and ranges of adaptive responses

Participants	Intervention phases				
	A	B	B'	A	B'
Adam	4 (3-5)	17.857 (10-22)	34.9 (23-48)	6.2 (5-7)	39 (25-48)
Brian	7 (4-8)	21.904 (14-28)	45.935 (25-56)	13.875 (10-19)	44.095 (28-57)

Table 2. Mean values and ranges of challenging behavior

Participants	Intervention phases				
	A	B	B'	A	B'
Adam	4 (3-5)	8.476 (6-15)	2.3 (1-6)	5.8 (5-6)	2.3 (1-5)
Brian	7 (4-9)	11.666 (10-15)	4.064 (1-9)	11.5 (6-16)	3.285 (1-6)

Table 3. Mean percentages and ranges of intervals with indices of positive participation

Participants	Intervention phases				
	A	B	B'	A	B'
Adam	5.2 (4-7)	24.285 (14-29)	31.7 (28-36)	9.8 (8-12)	28.45 (18-34)
Brian	8 (6-10)	22.666 (14-29)	31.129 (26-36)	9.625 (6-14)	32.666 (20-38)

4. DISCUSSION

Data largely supported previous empirical evidences [21-22-23] regarding the use of assistive technology-based programs to promote adaptive responses in children with FXS and multiple disabilities. Additionally, the study provided practical evidence of its beneficial effects on stereotypical behaviors and positive participation. Both participants significantly improved their performance during the intervention and cluster phases compared to the baseline. The rehabilitation program had positive outcomes on the quality of life of the participants involved [24-

25]. These results were consistent with the available literature [26-27-28] and suggested the following considerations.

First, the current investigation can be viewed as a profitable extension of previous findings focused on learning new adaptive responses and reducing stereotypic behaviors in children with FXS. It can also be considered effective in promoting self-determination and independence of the participants involved. Indeed, the AT program allowed participants to autonomously access positive stimulation. At the same time, they participated positively and increased their active role towards their environment by preventing their isolation and passivity, with beneficial outcomes for their social image, desirability, and status as they were constructively involved [29-30].

Second, technological supports can be considered as a great educational and rehabilitative resource for children with FXS and multiple disabilities, who commonly presented no interaction with the surrounding world, within home, medical, and school settings, with negative consequences on their social image and desirability [31]. Thus, such assistive technology may constitute an important way to support and eventually integrate parents, caregivers and teacher's mediation by reducing their burden [32]. Additionally, such approach may increase children's opportunities to have an active role in choices, and support self-determination [33-34-35]. In fact, AT can be considered an easy, simple and realistic or practical solution for complex clinical conditions. Thus, the management of two dependent variables (i. e., both adaptive response and challenging behavior), the provision of contingent stimulation (i.e., simultaneous presence of an adaptive response and absence of a challenging behavior), and the interruption of it whenever the challenging behavior occurred may be uneasy and / or onerous for parents and caregivers to be implemented.

Third, the technology may be viewed as a basic resource that could be updated and/or further extended, adapting it to participants' characteristics and learning capacities.

Thus, based on participants' progress and on daily contexts objectives (e.g., within school and home settings), one may envisage a third container facilitating the stimulation and the response variations. Moreover, one may design a microswitch cluster-based program, pursuing the dual objective of reinforcing an adaptive response and decreasing a challenging behavior such as hand mouthing and/or eye poking exhibited by Bernard and Adam. Participants would consequently learn self-control [36-37].

Fourth, the success of an MCT widely relied on the motivating potential of the delivered positive stimulation, the simplicity (i.e., low cost of response because already available in the behavioral repertoire), the manageability of the challenging behavior, and the suitability of the devices used. With regard to the first point, strong (i.e., highly rewarding) environmental events may profitably compensate the response cost. With regard to the second point, an easily reproducible adaptive response may be considered as crucial for the learning process. With regard to the third point, the manageability of the challenging behavior largely depends on the rapidity with it may be corrected and/ or redirected by or into a new adaptive response. With regard to the fourth point, the suitability of the devices used can be assessed with an easy matching between the adopted microswitches and the targeted responses/behaviors [38] The data of the current investigation suggested a favorable outcome with regard to each of the four aforementioned points.

Fifth, the use of such technological supports may be functional enabling Adam and Bernard to enrich their sensorial inputs with positive consequences on their mood. In fact, both increased their indices of positive participation during intervention and cross experimental phases. One may argue that both participants augmented their general sense of satisfaction and amount of pleasure, enjoying the sessions, and were positively involved. That is, by varying the responses and the environmental consequences they could prevent the saturation and increase their well-being [39-41].

5. LIMITATIONS

Despite the above discussed positive outcomes, this study presented some limitations. These data indicated that assistive technology-based program could support children with FXS and multiple disabilities, enabling them an active role, constructive engagement, occupation, and choice abilities. Undoubtedly, caution is needed considering that this a single-case design involving two participants, keeping in mind generalization limits. [42].

Furthermore, a functional analysis of the challenging behavior would be useful [43-44]. The current study was focused on basic and simple responses. Different and more sophisticated behavioral responses could be trained for the future. A systematic comparison with other behavioral interventions (e.g., differential or non-contingent reinforcements) would be useful (i.e., one delivered via microswitch and one administered via caregiver).

CONCLUSION AND FUTURE PERSPECTIVES

Future research perspectives in this area should deal with the following topics: (a) further extension of the assistive technology-based programs to other participants with FXS, adopting other behavioral responses and/or supplementary materials/activities (e.g., different objects in order to determine the external validity and the generalizability of the results), (b) updating the technology available and adapting it to a larger number of participants with FXS or other/different pathologies, and multiple disabilities with greater positive and beneficial effects [45-46]. Finally, one may envisage a social validation assessment, involving caregivers, parents, and teachers as raters [47].

REFERENCES

[1] Moskowitz LJ, Jones EA. Uncovering the evidence for behavioral interventions with individuals with fragile X syndrome: A systematic review. *Research in Developmental Disabilities*. 2015: 38: 223-241.

[2] Hagerman RJ, Polussa J. Treatment of the psychiatric problems associated with fragile X syndrome. *Current Opinion in Psychiatry*. 2015: 28(2): 107-112.

[3] Tonnsen BL, Grefer ML, Hatton DD, Roberts JE. Developmental trajectories of attentional control in preschool males with fragile X syndrome. *Research in Developmental Disabilities*. 2015: 36: 62-71.

[4] Stasolla F, Perilli V, Boccasini A. Assistive Technologies for Persons with Severe-Profound Intellectual and Developmental Disabilities In: *Computer-Assisted and Web-Based Innovations in Psychology, Special Education, and Health*. 2016; 287-310.

[5] Belva BC, & Matson JL. An examination of specific daily living skills deficits in adults with profound intellectual disabilities. *Research in Developmental Disabilities*. 2013: 34: 596–604.

[6] Chantry J, & Dunford C. How do computer assistive technologies enhance participation in childhood occupations for children with multiple and complex disabilities? A review of the current literature. *British Journal of Occupation Therapy*. 2010: 73, 351–365.

[7] Lancioni GE, & Singh NN. *Assistive technologies for people with diverse abilities*. New York: Springer. 2014.

[8] Matter R, Harniss M, Oderud T, Borg J, Eide AH. Assistive technology in resource-limited environments: A scoping review. *Disability and Rehabilitation on Assistive Technology*. 2017: 12: 105-14. PMID: 27443790.

[9] Lancioni GE, Singh NN, O'Reilly MF, Sigafoos J, Alberti G, Perilli V, Groeneweg J. People with multiple disabilities learn to engage in occupation and work activities with the support of technology-aided programs. *Research in Developmental Disabilities*. 2014; 35, 1264–1271.

[10] Stasolla F, & Perilli V. Microswitch-based programs (MBP) to promote communication, occupation, and leisure skills for children with multiple disabilities: A literature overview. In N. Silton (Ed.), *Recent advances in assistive technologies to support children with developmental disorders.* Hershey: IGI Global. 2015.

[11] Lancioni GE, Sigafoos J, O'Reilly MF, & Singh NN. Assistive technology. In *Interventions for individual with severe/profound and multiple disabilities.* New York: Springer. 2012.

[12] Stasolla F, Boccasini A, Perilli, V. Assistive technology-based programs to support adaptive behaviors by children with autism spectrum disorders: A literature overview. In Y. Kats (Ed.). *Supporting the education of children with autism spectrum disorders.* Hershey:IGI Global. 2016.

[13] Perrilli V, Stasolla F, Caffò AO, Albano V, D'Amico F. Microswitch-Cluster Technology for Promoting Occupation and Reducing Hand Biting of Six Adolescents with Fragile X Syndrome: New Evidence and Social Rating. *Journal of Developmental and Physical Disabilities.* 2018.

[14] Stasolla F, Perilli V, Damiani R, Albano V. Assistive technology to promote occupation and reduce mouthing by three boys with fragile X syndrome. *Developmental Neurorehabilitation.* 2016: 7: 1-9.

[15] Stasolla F, Perilli V, Caffò AO, Boccasini A, Stella A, Damiani R. Extending microswitch-cluster programs to promote occupation activities and reduce mouthing by six children with autism spectrum disorders and intellectual disabilities. *Journal of Developmental and Physical Disabilities.* 2017: 29: 307–324.

[16] Wilkinson KM, Hennig S. The state of research and practice in augmentative and alternative communication for children with developmental/intellectual disabilities. *Mental Retardation and Developmental Disabilities Research.* 2007: 13: 58-69.

[17] Mirrett PL, Roberts JE, Price J. Early intervention practices and communication intervention strategies for young males with fragile X syndrome. *Language, Speech, and Hearing Services in Schools.* 2003: 34: 320–331.

[18] Crawford MR, Schuster JW. Using microswitches to teach toy use. *Journal of Developmental and Physical Disabilities*. 1993: 5: 349–368.

[19] Stasolla F, Perilli V, Caffò AO, Boccasini A, Stella A, Damiani R. . Extending microswitch-cluster programs to promote occupation activities and reduce mouthing by six children with autism spectrum disorders and intellectual disabilities. *Journal of Developmental and Physical Disabilities*. 2017: 29: 307–324.

[20] Barlow DH, Nock M, Hersen M. *Single-case experimental designs: Strategies for studying behavior changes*. New York: Allyn & Bacon. 2009.

[21] Lancioni GE, O'Reilly MF, Campodonico F. Technological resources to support adaptive responding with persons with multiple disabilities. *Scandinavian Journal of Behavior Therapy*. 2001: 30: 17–22.

[22] Lancioni GE, Singh NN, O'Reilly MF, Sigafoos J, Alberti G, Perilli V. People with multiple disabilities learn to engage in occupation and work activities with the support of technology-aided programs. *Research in Developmental Disabilities*: 2014: 35: 1264–1271.

[23] Shih CH, Chang ML. A wireless object location detector enabling people with developmental disabilities to control environmental stimulation through simple occupation activities with Nintendo Wij balance boards. *Research in Developmental Disabilities*. 2012: 33: 983–989.

[24] Felce D, Perry J. Quality of life: Its definition and measurement. *Research in Developmental Disabilities*. 1995: 16: 51–74.

[25] Stasolla, F, Damiani R, Caffo` AO. Promoting constructive engagement by two boys with autism spectrum disorders and high functioning through behavioral interventions. *Research in Autism Spectrum Disorders*. 2014: 8: 376–380.

[26] Budimirovic DB, Berry-Kravis E, Erickson CA, Hall SS, Hessl D, Reiss AL. Updated report on tools to measure outcomes of clinical trials in fragile X syndrome. *Journal of Neurodevelopmental Disorders*. 2017: 9(1): 14.

[27] Hare EB, Hagerman RJ, Lozano R. Targeted treatments in fragile X syndrome. *Expert Opinion on Orphan Drugs*. 2014: 2: 531–543.

[28] Fisch GS, Carpenter N, Howard-Peebles PN, Holden JJA, Tarleton J, Simensen R, Battaglia A. Developmental trajectories in syndromes with intellectual disability, with a focus on wolf- Hirschhorn and its cognitive behavioral profile. *American Journal on Intellectual and Developmental Disabilities*. 2012: 117: 167–179.

[29] Chiapparino C, Stasolla F, de Pace C, Lancioni GE. A touch pad and a scanning keyboard emulator to facilitate writing by a woman with extensive motor disability. *Life Span and Disability*. 2011: 14: 45–54.

[30] Stasolla F, & De Pace C. Assistive technology to promote leisure and constructive engagement by two boys emerged from a minimal conscious state. *Neurorehabilitation*. 2014: 35: 253–259.

[31] McDougall J, Evans J, Baldwin P. The importance of self-determination to perceived quality of life for youth and young adults with chronic conditions and disabilities. *Remedial and Special Education*. 2010: 31: 252–260.

[32] Lancioni GE, Singh NN. *Assistive technologies for people with diverse abilities*. New York: Springer. 2014.

[33] Stasolla F, De Pace C. Assistive technology to promote leisure and constructive engagement by two boys emerged from a minimal conscious state. *Neuro Rehabilitation*. In press: 7-10.

[34] Stasolla F, Caffo` AO. Promoting adaptive behaviors by two girls with Rett syndrome through a microswich-based program. *Research in Autism Spectrum Disorders*. 2013: 7: 1265–1272.

[35] Tullis CA, Cannella-Malone HI, Basbigill AR, Yeager A, Fleming CV, Payne D. Review of the choice and preference assessment literature for individuals with severe to profound disabilities. *Education and Training in Autism and Developmental Disabilities*. 2011: 46: 576–595.

[36] Stasolla F, Perilli V, Damiani R, Caffo` AO, Di Leone A, Albano V. A microswitch cluster program to enhance object manipulation and to reduce hand mouthing by three children with autism spectrum

disorders and intellectual disabilities. *Research in Autism Spectrum Disorders*. 2014: 8: 1071–1078.

[37] Tureck K, Matson JL, Beighley JS. An investigation of self-injurious behaviours in adults with severe intellectual disabilities. *Research in Developmental Disabilities*. 2013: 34: 2469–2474.

[38] Lancioni GE, Singh NN, O'Reilly MF, Sigafoos J, Alberti G, Perilli V, Groeneweg J. People with multiple disabilities learn to engage in occupation and work activities with the support of technology-aided programs. *Research in Developmental Disabilities*. 2014: 35: 1264–1271.

[39] Catania AC. *Learning* (5th ed.). New York: Sloan. 2015.

[40] Dillon CM, Carr JE. Assessing indices of happiness and unhappiness in individuals with developmental disabilities: A review. *Behavioural Interventions*. 2007: 22: 229–244.

[41] Lancioni GE, Singh NN, O'Reilly MF, Sigafoos J, Chiapparino C, Stasolla F. Using an optic sensor and a scanning keyboard emulator to facilitate writing by persons with pervasive motor disabilities. *Journal of Developmental and Physical Disabilities*. 2007: 19: 593–603.

[42] Kennedy CH. *Single-case designs for educational research*. Boston: Allyn & Bacon. 2005.

[43] Hardiman RL, McGill P. The topographies and operant functions of challenging behaviours in fragile X syndrome: A systematic review and analysis of existing data. *Journal of Intellectual and Developmental Disability*. 2017: 42: 190–203.

[44] Machalicek W, McDuffie A, Oakes A, Ma M, Thurman AJ, Rispoli MJ, Abbeduto L. Examining the operant function of challenging behavior in young males with fragile X syndrome: A summary of 12 cases. *Research in Developmental Disabilities*. 2014: 35: 1694–1704.

[45] Matson JL, Cervantes PE. Comorbidity among persons with intellectual disabilities. *Research in Autism Spectrum Disorders*. 2013: 7: 1318–1322.

[46] Naslund R, Gardelli A. "I know, I can, I will try": Youths and adults with intellectual disabilities in Sweden using information and communication technology in their everyday life. *Disability and Society*. 2013: 28: 28–40.

[47] Scherer MJ, Craddock G, Mackeogh T. The relationship of personal factors and subjective well-being to the use of assistive technology devices. *Disability and Rehabilitation*. 2011: 33: 811–817.

In: Fragile X Syndrome
Editor: Fabrizio Stasolla

ISBN: 978-1-68507-572-9
© 2022 Nova Science Publishers, Inc.

Chapter 6

MICROSWITCH AND VOCA TO INDEPENDENTLY ACCESS POSITIVE STIMULATION AND ASK FOR SOCIAL INTERACTION IN AN ADOLESCENT WITH FRAGILE X SYNDROME AND DEVELOPMENTAL DISABILITIES

Fabrizio Stasolla[1,*], Donatella Ciarmoli[1]
and Vincenza Albano[2]

[1]"Giustino Fortunato" University of Benevento (Italy)
[2]Department of Educational Sciences, Psychology, Communication,
University "Aldo Moro" of Bari (Italy)

---

[*]Corresponding Author's E-mail: f.stasolla@unifortunato.eu.

ABSTRACT

Background

Individuals with Fragile X syndrome may have intellectual, motor, and communication impairments with few opportunities to positively access to pleasant stimuli or ask for social interaction with a caregiver.

Objectives

To provide an adolescent with Fragile X syndrome and severe to profound developmental disabilities with an independent access to positive stimulation and social interaction with his parents.

Method

A combined microswitch and VOCA rehabilitative program was implemented. A multiple probe design was adopted. An assistive technology-based intervention was proposed.

Results

Data evidenced that the participant profitably learned the functional use of the technology and was enabled to positive stimulation and ensured with social interactions.

Conclusion

An assistive technology-based program was helpful to promote the active role and constructive engagement of an adolescent with Fragile X syndrome and developmental disabilities.

Keywords: assistive technology, quality of life, constructive engagement, social interactions, independence

1. INTRODUCTION

Fragile X syndrome is a genetic disease due to an excessive length of the repetitive sequence of trinucleotides (CGG) in the FMR1 gene, located on the long arm of X chromosome [1-3]. It constitutes one of the most inherited causes of severe to profound developmental disabilities, motor delays, and communicative impairments [4-5]. Next to learning difficulties, challenging behaviors, epilepsy, attention deficits and hyperactivity disorders may be frequently acknowledged. Furthermore, aggression and self-injury behaviors (SIB) are observed. Hand biting and mouthing stereotypic behaviors are additionally included [6]. Narrow face, large head and ears, flexible joints, flat feet, and prominent forehead are commonly included in the phenotype [7-8]. Anxiety, trouble with gaze contact, difficulties in verbal communication, and sensorial hyper-sensibility are finally embedded [9-10].

Children and adolescents with FXS may pose serious challenges to daily rehabilitative centers due their clinical conditions, which preclude an active role, communication interactions, constructive engagement, and positive participation to social life [11]. Thus, that situation may seriously hamper their social image, desirability, and status with negative outcomes on their quality of life. To overcome this issue, one may rely on assistive technology-based interventions (AT) [11-12]. AT refers to any piece, device, equipment or tool capable of minimizing the existing gap between the behavioral repertoire and environmental requests. Accordingly, an individual with multiple disabilities will be ensured with an active role, self-determination, positive participation, and constructive engagement towards everyday life requests [13-15]. A basic form of AT is represented by microswitches [16].

Microswitches are electronic tools which provide the independent access to positive stimulation in individuals with multiple disabilities. That is, through small behavioral responses, an individual with multiple disabilities might activate brief periods of positive stimulation via technological systems, control system unit, and adapted software [16]. For example, a boy diagnosed with cerebral palsy and extensive motor impairments may be provided with 7 seconds of positive stimulation through arms and/or legs movements [17]. Unfortunately, a microswitch-based programs (MBP) is limited to such access because it does not provide the individual with social interaction [18]. The latter objective may be pursued through a vocal output communication aid (VOCA) device, which represents a communication tool capable of ensuring the individual with social interaction. Thus, by selecting a non-verbal, behavioral response, the participant with multiple disabilities will be enabled to ask the social interaction with a caregiver [19-20]. Combined with a MBP, a VOCA device may represent a rehabilitative option in which the participant may choose whether independently access to positive stimulation (i.e., microswitch selection) or ask for the social interaction with a caregiver [21]. Although the literature on that combination is robust, no studies have been carried out with FXS participants [22].

Accordingly with the above, the current chapter pursued the following objectives: (a) to include an adolescent with FXS in a combined rehabilitative program with microswitch and VOCA options, (b) to enable the participant with independent access to positive stimulation, (c) to ensure the participant with the opportunity of social interactions, and (d) to provide the participant with choice options between both solutions.

2. METHOD

2.1. Participant and Setting

George was a 15-years old adolescent diagnosed with FXS from DNA results and laboratory tests, at the beginning of the study. His intellectual functioning assessed through the Vineland Assessment Behavioral Scale (VABS-II) administrated by his psychologist revealed an intellectual age of 1.5 years. He presented severe to profound developmental disabilities, although he was capable of few adaptive behavioral responses through object manipulation and head-side turning. He attended regular classes with a support teacher and a special education program 18 hours per week.

He was unable to verbal speech, sphincteric control, and presented seizures, anxiety, and aggression, as described by their parents and caregivers. Furthermore, their teachers reported that he was capable of adaptive responding whenever involved in functional activities and was constructively engaged accordingly. He evidenced hand-mouthing related stereotypy as part of his behavioral repertoire. He was additionally described as quite isolated and passive, although he participated to speech and physiotherapy sessions three days per week.

Their parents found the MBP program combined with a VOCA highly promising and were enthusiastic to be involved in the program itself. In fact, they signed a formal consent for the inclusion of George in the program, which was approved by a local ethic and scientific committee. The study was carried out in the participant's home in a silent room preserved from any external or environmental interference.

2.2. Technology and Responses

The adaptive responses consisted in object manipulation (i.e., microswitch activation), and head-left turning (i.e., VOCA activation). The adapted microswitches consisted in a wobble (i.e., a ball-like pressure microswitch which needed to be pulled, pushed, or moved side-way to be activated), and a tilt sensor for the microswitch and VOCA activations, respectively. The technology additionally included a control system unit with an adapted software capable of managing both responses and activations. Finally, the system control unit automatically delivered the positive stimulation during intervention phases (i.e., see experimental conditions below).

2.3. Preference Screening

Beside an informal interview with parents and caregivers, a formal preference screening occurred [23]. Thus, six 5-min sessions were collected. Ten seconds of stimulus presentation were alternated with 15-20 seconds rest intervals by two research assistants who noted the participants' reactions according to three basic criteria, namely (a) alert, (b) orientation, and (c) smiling. Stimuli preferred by George according to one or more of the aforementioned criteria at least in the 80% of the presentations were retained as positive and primary reinforcers. George was amused by selected songs, colored lights, and tactile vibrations.

Furthermore, his parents preliminarily recorded brief verbal messages enabling social interactions. That messages, systematically varied to prevent saturation, were used during VOCA intervention sessions [24].

2.4. Sessions and Data Collections

The study lasted three months. Typically, three 5-min sessions were collected 5 days per week. Overall, 180 sessions were carried out. Data collection included (a) microswitch activations (i.e., wobble activations), and VOCA activations (i.e., tilt activations), according to an event recording coding system [25].

2.5. Experimental Conditions

The study was conducted according to a multiple probe single-subject experimental design [26], in which subsequently to a baseline on both adaptive responses, each adaptive response was first learned singly and consolidated before being combined with the other. A choice opportunity was ensured accordingly.

2.5.1. First Baseline
During the initial baseline, the technology was available but inactive. Thus, even if an adaptive response occurred, no environmental consequences were provided. Ten sessions were collected on both adaptive responses along three days.

2.5.2. First Intervention

During the first intervention, focused on microswitch activations, each object manipulation, detected through the wobble microswitch was contingently reinforced with 6 seconds of positive stimulation (i.e., preferred songs, colored lights, and tactile vibrations). Reinforcers were automatically and systematically varied throughout the sessions. Forty sessions were collected along three weeks.

2.5.3. Second Baseline

Once the learning process was consolidated on microswitch responding, a new baseline occurred on VOCA activations. Conditions were identical to the first baseline and ten sessions were conducted along three days.

2.5.4. Second Intervention

During the second intervention, VOCA responses were targeted. Thus, each left head- turning detected through the tilt microswitch fixed on a hat produced a brief vocal message asking for social interaction. Accordingly, George's mother or father positively interacted with their son contingently to the participant's adaptive responding. Forty sessions were conducted along three weeks. During such phase, the intervention on microswitch responding (i.e., first adaptive response of object manipulation) was suspended.

2.5.5. Third Intervention

Once consolidated the second adaptive (i.e., VOCA) response, a combined intervention occurred. George was equipped with both devices and was free to choose whether activate the wobble or the tilt devices. Whenever the participant activated the wobble, he received 6 sec of positive stimulation. Conversely, if the boy activated the tilt, he was enabled with social interaction. Eighty sessions were collected along two months.

3. RESULTS

Data were summarized in Table 1.

Table 1. Data summary grouped according to experimental conditions

A	B	A	B	C
3-5	22	4	15	18-12

Table 1 summarizes mean values of adaptive responses along the experimental phases. During the initial baseline, the mean value of microswitch responding was 3 (range 1-4), while the mean value of VOCA adaptive responding was 5 (range 3-7). During the first intervention, George increased his adaptive responding up to 22 (mean value, with a range comprised between 16 and 27). Along the second baseline, the participant produced 4 VOCA activations (range 3-5), indicating that both behaviors were independent one to each other. Along the second intervention phase, the adolescent improved his adaptive responding with an increased performance up to 15 (range 12-19). Finally, along the combined phase, George evidenced a functional use of both devices and related options, with a mean value of 18 (range 14-21), and 12 (range (10-15) for microswitch and VOCA activations, respectively. The Kolmogorov-Smirnov test revealed that differences between the experimental phases were significant ($p < .01$).

4. DISCUSSION

Collected data showed that the MBP combined with a VOCA option was effective and suitable to promote an active role, constructive engagement, social interaction, and positive participation in an adolescent with FXS and developmental delays. George improved his adaptive responding and emphasized that his active role and constructive engagement were purposeful. Findings were consistent with the existing literature [27-30] and suggested some considerations.

First, an AT-based intervention was useful to help an individual with FXS in adaptive responding. Thus, George was ensured with independent access to positive participation. Moreover, his constructive engagement was corroborated. His motivation was promoted and his positive occupation enhanced. George was constructively engaged and his functional participation prevented isolation, withdrawal, and passivity. That access was additionally helpful to reduce parents' burden [31-32].

Second, the opportunity of social interaction with his parents was fostered. Thus, George was enabled to receive tangible items or personal needs mediated by his parents. Isolation was further avoided because he could socially interact with his family and reach pleasant stimulation at the same time [33-34].

Third, the multiple probe experimental design provided George with choice options. Thus, during the final intervention phases, he could select alternatively a behavioral response and activate the related technological device to get access to one environmental event or a second consequence instead. One may argue that the provision of inputs was meaningfully enriched [35-36].

CONCLUSION

Despite the encouraging and promising results, the current investigations highlighted some limitations to be addressed in future empirical contributions. First, it was a single-subject case report with a unique adolescent as participant. Accordingly, caution was undoubtedly mandatory. Second, an outcome measure of the participant's quality of life (e.g., indices of happiness or positive participation) was currently missing and should be considered. Third, the preference checks to investigate whether the participant preferred the microswitch or VOCA activations should be included. Follow-up, maintenance or generalization phases were not assessed. Finally, social validation procedures including external raters should be evaluated.

In light of the above, future research perspectives should deal with the following topics (a) extension to additional participants with FXS and developmental disabilities, (b) extension to new adaptive responses and new adapted microswitches or technological devices, (c) a participant' preference assessment, and (d) social validation procedures including different groups of external raters [37].

REFERENCES

[1] Lang, S; Bartl-Pokorny, KD; Pokorny, FB; Garrido, D; Mani, N; Fox-Boyer, AV; et al. Canonical Babbling: A Marker for Earlier Identification of Late Detected Developmental Disorders? *Curr Develop Disord Rep*, 2019, 6(3), 111-118.

[2] Purugganan, O. Intellectual disabilities. *Pediatr Rev*, 2018, 39(6), 299-309.

[3] Morel, A; Peyroux, E; Leleu, A; Favre, E; Franck, N; Demily, C. Overview of social cognitive dysfunctions in rare developmental syndromes with psychiatric phenotype. *Front Pediatr*, 2018, 6.

[4] Fernandez, BA; Scherer, SW. Syndromic autism spectrum disorders: Moving from a clinically defined to a molecularly defined approach. *Dialogues Clin Neurosci*, 2017, 19(4), 353-371.

[5] Glennon, JM; Karmiloff-Smith, A; Thomas, MSC. Syndromic Autism: Progressing Beyond Current Levels of Description. *Rev J Autism Dev Disord*, 2017, 4(4), 321-327.

[6] Man, L; Lekovich, J; Rosenwaks, Z; Gerhardt, J. Fragile X-associated diminished ovarian reserve and primary ovarian insufficiency from molecular mechanisms to clinical manifestations. *Front Mol Neurosci*, 2017, 10.

[7] Smith, MG; Royer, J; Mann, J; McDermott, S; Valdez, R. Capture-recapture methodology to study rare conditions using surveillance

data for fragile X syndrome and muscular dystrophy. *Orphanet J Rare Dis*, 2017, 12(1).

[8] Wang, JY; Ngo, MM; Hessl, D; Hagerman, RJ; Rivera, SM. Robust machine learning-based correction on automatic segmentation of the cerebellum and brainstem. *PLoS ONE*, 2016, 11(5).

[9] Zuo, L; Tan, Y; Wang, Z; Wang, K; Zhang, X; Chen, X; et al. Long noncoding RNAs in psychiatric disorders. *Psychiatr Genet*, 2016, 26(3), 109-116.

[10] Fraint, A; Vittal, P; Szewka, A; Bernard, B; Berry-Kravis, E; Hall, DA. New observations in the fragile X-associated tremor/ataxia syndrome (FXTAS) phenotype. *Front Genet*, 2014, 5(SEP).

[11] Riley, K; Bodine, C; Hills, J; Gane, LW; Sandstrum, J; Hagerman, R. The tickle box assistive technology device piloted on a young woman with fragile X syndrome. *Ment Health Asp Dev Disabil*, 2001, 4(4), 138-142.

[12] Mirrett, PL; Roberts, JE; Price, J. Early Intervention Practices and Communication Intervention Strategies for Young Males with Fragile X Syndrome. *Lang Speech Hear Serv Sch*, 2003, 34(4), 320-331.

[13] Stasolla, F; Boccasini, A; Perilli, V; Caffò, AO; Damiani, R; Albano, V. A selective overview of microswitch-based programs for promoting adaptive behaviors of children with developmental disabilities. *Int J Ambient Comput Intell*, 2014, 6(2), 56-74.

[14] Stasolla, F; Perilli, V; Boccasini, A; Caffò, AO; Damiani, R; Albano, V. Enhancing academic performance of three boys with autism spectrum disorders and intellectual disabilities through a computer-based program. *Life Span Disabil*, 2016,19(2),153-183.

[15] Stasolla, F; Perilli, V; Caffò, AO; Boccasini, A; Stella, A; Damiani, R; et al. Extending microswitch-cluster programs to promote occupation activities and reduce mouthing by six children with autism spectrum disorders and intellectual disabilities. *J Dev Phys Disabil*, 2017, 29(2), 307-324.

[16] Stasolla, F; Caffò, AO; Perilli, V; Boccasini, A; Stella, A; Damiani, R; et al. a microswitch-based program for promoting initial

ambulation responses: An evaluation with two girls with multiple disabilities. *J Appl Behav Anal*, 2017, 50(2), 345-356.

[17] Lancioni, GE; O'Reilly, MF; Singh, NN; Stasolla, F; Manfredi, F; Oliva, D. Adapting a grid into a microswitch to suit simple hand movements of a child with profound multiple disabilities. *Percept Mot Skills*, 2004, 99(2), 724-728.

[18] Lancioni, GE; Singh, NN; O'Reilly, MF; Sigafoos, J; Ricci, I; Addante, LM; et al. A woman with multiple disabilities uses a VOCA system to request for and access caregiver-mediated stimulation events. *Life Span Disabil*, 2011, 14(2), 91-99.

[19] Lancioni, GE; O'Reilly, MF; Singh, NN; Sigafoos, J; Didden, R; Oliva, D; et al. Persons with multiple disabilities accessing stimulation and requesting social contact via microswitch and VOCA devices: New research evaluation and social validation. *Res Dev Disabil*, 2009, 30(5), 1084-1094.

[20] Lancioni, GE; O'Reilly, MF; Singh, N; Sigafoos, J; Oliva, D; Smaldone, A; et al. Persons with multiple disabilities access stimulation and contact the caregiver via microswitch and VOCA technology. *Life Span Disabil*, 2009, 12(2), 119-128.

[21] Lancioni, GE; O'Reilly, MF; Cuvo, AJ; Singh, NN; Sigafoos, J; Didden, R. PECS and VOCAs to enable students with developmental disabilities to make requests: An overview of the literature. *Res Dev Disabil*, 2007, 28(5), 468-488.

[22] Lancioni, GE; Singh, NN; O'Reilly, MF; Sigafoos, J; Alberti, G; Perilli, V; et al. Microswitch-aided programs to support physical exercise or adequate ambulation in persons with multiple disabilities. *Res Dev Disabil*, 2014, 35(9), 2190-2198.

[23] Crawford, MR; Schuster, JW. Using microswitches to teach toy use. *J Dev Phys Disabil*, 1993, 5(4), 349-368.

[24] Lancioni, GE; O'Reilly, MF; Cuvo, AJ; Singh, NN; Sigafoos, J; Didden, R. PECS and VOCAs to enable students with developmental disabilities to make requests: An overview of the literature. *Res Dev Disabil*, 2007, 28(5), 468-488.

[25] Stasolla, F; Caffò, AO; Ciarmoli, D; Albano, V. Promoting Object Manipulation and Reducing Tongue Protrusion in Seven Children with Angelman Syndrome and Developmental Disabilities through Microswitch-Cluster Technology: a Research Extension. *J Dev Phys Disabil*, 2021, 33(5), 799-817.

[26] Stasolla, F; Caffò, AO; Damiani, R; Perilli, V; Di Leone A; Albano V. Assistive technology-based programs to promote communication and leisure activities by three children emerged from a minimal conscious state. *Cogn Process*, 2015, 16(1), 69-78.

[27] Stasolla, F; Perilli, V; Damiani, R; Albano, V. Assistive technology to promote occupation and reduce mouthing by three boys with fragile X syndrome. *Dev Neurorehabilitation*, 2017, 20(4), 185-193.

[28] Stasolla, F; Perilli, V; Damiani, R; Albano, V. Assistive technology to promote occupation and reduce mouthing by three boys with fragile X syndrome. *Dev Neurorehabilitation*, 2017, 20(4), 185-193.

[29] Robb, N; Northridge, J; Politis, Y; Zhang, B. Parental intention to support the use of computerized cognitive training for children with genetic neurodevelopmental disorders. *Front Public Health*, 2018, 6.

[30] Riley, K; Bodine, C; Hills, J; Gane, LW; Sandstrum, J; Hagerman, R. The tickle box assistive technology device piloted on a young woman with fragile X syndrome. *Ment Health Asp Dev Disabil*, 2001, 4(4), 138-142.

[31] Bharucha, AJ; Anand, V; Forlizzi, J; Dew, MA; Reynolds, CF; Stevens, S; et al. Intelligent assistive technology applications to dementia care: Current capabilities, limitations, and future challenges. *Am J Geriatr Psychiatry*, 2009, 17(2), 88-104.

[32] Robb, N; Northridge, J; Politis, Y; Zhang, B. Parental intention to support the use of computerized cognitive training for children with genetic neurodevelopmental disorders. *Front Public Health*, 2018, 6.

[33] Freda, MF; Savarese, L; Bova, M; Galante, A; De Falco, R; De Luca Picione, R; et al. Stress and Psychological Factors in the Variable Clinical Phenotype of Hereditary Angioedema in Children: A Pilot Study. *Pediatr Allergy Immunol Pulmonol*, 2016, 29(1), 6-12.

[34] Dicé, F; Auricchio, M; Boursier, V; De Luca Picione, R; Santamaria, F; Salerno, M; et al. Psychological Scaffolding for taking charge of Intersex/DSD conditions. The Joint Listening Settings. *Psicol Salute*, 2018, 2018(1), 129-145.

[35] Stasolla, F; Caffò, AO; Perilli, V; Boccasini, A; Damiani, R; D'Amico, F. Assistive technology for promoting adaptive skills of children with cerebral palsy: ten cases evaluation. *Disabil Rehabil Assistive Technol*, 2019, 14(5), 489-502.

[36] Stasolla, F; Damiani, R; Perilli, V; D'Amico, F; Caffò, AO; Stella, A; et al. Computer and microswitch-based programs to improve academic activities by six children with cerebral palsy. *Res Dev Disabil*, 2015, 45-46, 1-13.

[37] Lancioni, GE; O'Reilly, MF; Singh, NN; Groeneweg, J; Bosco, A; Tota, A; et al. A social validation assessment of microswitch-based programs for persons with multiple disabilities employing teacher trainees and parents as raters. *J Dev Phys Disabil*, 2006, 18(4), 383-391.

In: Fragile X Syndrome
Editor: Fabrizio Stasolla

ISBN: 978-1-68507-572-9
© 2022 Nova Science Publishers, Inc.

Chapter 7

PROMOTING FUNCTIONAL OCCUPATION IN A CHILD WITH FRAGILE X SYNDROME: EFFECTS ON POSITIVE MOOD

Fabrizio Stasolla[1,*], *Vincenza Albano*[2] *and Donatella Ciarmoli*[1]

[1]Giustino Fortunato University of Benevento, Benevento, Italy
[2]Department of Educational Sciences, Psychology, Communication, Aldo Moro University of Bari, Bari, Italy

ABSTRACT

Background

Fragile X syndrome is an inherited disease and a basic cause of severe to profound developmental disabilities, with isolation and passivity commonly included as main features.

---

[*] Corresponding Author's E-mail: f.stasolla@uniforttunato.eu.

Objectives

To promote functional occupation in a boy with Fragile X syndrome. To evaluate an assistive technology-based program on indices of happiness as an outcome measure of the participant's quality of life.

Method

A cross-over single subject experimental design was implemented. The associations between behavioral responses and environmental consequences were systematically inverted.

Results

Data showed that the participant functionally acquired the awareness between the adaptive responding and the environmental consequences. The child increased the indices of happiness as well.

Conclusion

An assistive technology-based program was useful to promote positive occupation and increase indices of happiness in a child with Fragile X syndrome and developmental disabilities.

Keywords: fragile X syndrome, positive participation, indices of happiness, quality of life, assistive technology

1. INTRODUCTION

Fragile X syndrome (FXS) is an inherited disease caused by mutations in the FMR1 gene found on the X chromosome. The mutation affects how the body produces the Mental Retardation Protein or FMPR. The body makes only a little bit or none of the protein, which is the cause of symptoms in FXS. Developmental and intellectual disabilities are usually embedded. Learning difficulties, cognitive and behavioral problems are usually included [1-3]. The syndrome additionally hampers the child's development with negative outcomes on communication skills, physical appearance, sensitivity to noise, light and further sensory information [4, 5]. Anxiety, aggression, impulsivity, hyperactivity, and seizures are part of the syndrome [6]. Isolation, withdrawal, and passivity are additionally acknowledged, beside challenging (i.e., stereotypic, hand-related biting or mouthing) behaviors [7, 8]. To overcome this issue, which may be deleterious for the individual's quality of life, one may resort to assistive technology-based interventions (AT) and/or cognitive-behavioral programs [9, 10].

AT encompasses any piece, device, equipment, or tool designed to enhance the person's independence, self-determination, active role, and constructive engagement towards the outside world. Thus, AT is implemented to build a functional bridge capable of minimizing the distance between the individual behavioral repertoire and the environmental daily life requests [11, 12]. Consequently, the participant is enabled with positive participation, functional occupation, choice opportunities, communication skills, locomotion options, and constructive engagement in daily settings [13]. Furthermore, the participation may be promoted with both families and caregivers' burden reduction [14]. Because individuals with FXS are described as intellectual, motor, communicatively, and sensorially impaired, they can be considered individuals with multiple disabilities. That population may be equipped with microswitch-based programs (MBP) [15].

MBP are based on electronic tools (i.e., sensors) capable of detecting small behavioral responses ensuring the individual with brief periods of positive stimulation contingently, through an electronic system provided with a control unit [16]. Although the literature on the use of MBP in individuals with multiple disabilities is substantial, few studies have been conducted and assessed its effects in participants with FXS [17, 18].

Accordingly, the current investigation addressed the use of a MBP in a little boy with FXS and severe to profound developmental delays to promote occupation activities and evaluated the acquisition of the choice capacities. Moreover, it assessed the effects of such rehabilitative program on the participant's indices of happiness as an outcome measure of positive mood and an index of his quality of life [19, 20].

2. METHOD

2.1. Participant and Setting

Henry was a 5.5 boy diagnosed with FXS through laboratory test and DNA results. He was additionally mosaic because he presented the full gene mutation and premutation responsible for the FXS. The Vineland Adaptive Behavioral Scale (i.e., VABS - II) assessed by his psychologist, evidenced a chronological age of 1.2 years and indicated the participant as an individual with severe to profound developmental disabilities. He was reported by their parents as quite isolated and passive, and frequently exhibited withdrawal in daily activities. He showed lack of speech, hand-mouthing stereotypic behavior, lack of sphincter control, isolation, and passivity, beside anxiety and aggression. He attended regular classes with a special teacher and a specific educational program 24 hours per week. Nevertheless, he was capable of functional activities such as sorting objects whenever adequately rewarded and motivated.

His parents were favorable to an AT-based program and were enthusiastic to participate in such MBP proposal focused on promoting occupation and enhancing positive participation, next to constructive engagement. The study was conducted in a silent room of the participant's home. His parents signed as legal representatives a formal consent. The study was approved by a local ethic and scientific committee. Finally, the investigation was carried out according to Helsinki Declaration and its later amendments.

2.2. Technology and Response

The adaptive response consisted of sorting objects in a container. Specifically, Henry disposed of three rectangular containers in front of him (30 x 40 centimeters) equipped with two optic sensors (i.e., photocells). Additionally, each container was provided with a 9 x 13 centimeters' picture indicating bottles, cars, and toy soldiers, respectively. Henry disposed of such objects to be sorted in the correct container in each session (i.e., see below experimental conditions). Each optic sensor was connected with a laptop and a system control unit, fixed behind the containers, visible but inaccessible to the participant, which ensured the child with brief periods of positive stimulation, except for the baseline phases (see below, experimental conditions).

2.3. Preference Screening

Complimentary to an informal 30-minutes interview with both parents and teachers, a formal screening of positive stimulation was performed [21]. Thus, seven 5-minutes sessions were collected with 10 seconds of presentations alternated by 15-20 seconds of rest intervals by two research assistants. Stimuli positively appreciated by Henry according three basic criteria, namely (a) attention, (b) orientation, and (c) smiling were retained. Amusing songs, funny videos, and colored lights were selected as reinforcers to be used during intervention sessions (see below).

2.4. Sessions and Data Collection

The study lasted four months. Typically, three 5-minutes sessions were collected, four days per week. Data collection included (a) the sorted objected correctly inserted in each container and (b) indices of happiness (i.e., smiling, laughing, excited arms, legs, and body movements with or without vocalizations) according to a 15-seconds partial interval coding system. That is, 10 seconds of observation were followed by 5 seconds of dichotomous recording (i.e., absence or presence) as an index in the previous observed interval [22].

2.5. Inter-Rater Observation Agreement (IOA)

Two research assistants coded simultaneously and independently the sessions. An IOA percentage was calculated considering the number of agreements divided by the number of agreements added to the number of disagreements and multiplying it by 100 [23]. The mean percentage of agreement was 96 with a range comprised between 94 and 100%.

2.6. Experimental Conditions

The study was carried out according to a cross-over experimental design [24] in which the associations between the sorted objects with the positioned containers (i.e., on the participant' left, center, or right) and the environmental consequences (i.e., songs, videos, and/or lights) were randomly and systematically inverted to avoid saturation and enhance choice opportunities.

2.6.1. Baseline
During the baseline, the technology was available but inactive. The adaptive response (i.e., sorting objects) did not produce any environmental events. Overall, 15 sessions were collected along three baseline phases, considering the initial baseline and the following phases. The three baselines were completed within a week.

2.6.2. Intervention
During the three intervention phases, as detailed above, the associations between behavioral responses and environmental consequences were randomly inverted.

Thus, during the first intervention phase, the bottles container was on Henry's left, the cars container on his center, and the toy soldiers on his right. Five seconds of positive stimulation were automatically delivered. Thus, contingently Henry received 5 seconds of songs if he sorted a bottle, 5 seconds of lights were delivered if Henry sorted a car, and 5 seconds of videos were automatically delivered if Henry sorted a toy soldier. That association was systematically inverted to evaluate whether Henry acquired or not the awareness of the association along three intervention phases, which lasted three months.

3. RESULTS

Data were grouped over blocks of sessions and summarized in tables 1 and 2. Table 1 summarized the sorting objects adaptive response, and table 2 summarized the indices of happiness. Henry systematically varied his adaptive responding according to the inversion of the positioned containers and the environmental events, emphasizing his awareness. Additionally, indices of happiness varied according to the participant's preferences. The Kolmogorov-Smirnov test evidenced statistically significant differences ($p < .001$).

Table 1. Mean values of sorted objects according to the experimental phases

A	B	A	B	A	B	A	B
2	10	3	12	3	15	2	16
1	15	2	14	2	13	1	14
2	12	1	13	1	11	2	13

Table 2. Mean intervals with indices of happiness according to the experimental phases

A	B	A	B	A	B	A	B
5	16	4	17	3	18	2	14
4	15	3	16	2	16	3	15
3	13	4	14	1	17	2	18

4. DISCUSSION

Data showed that the MBP was helpful to increase the adaptive responding of the participant with FXS and developmental disabilities. The intervention improved the participant's adaptive responding, enhanced his opportunities of choices and promoted his positive mood. Henry was constructively engaged, positively occupied, and functionally active. The boy was capable of sorting objects and improved his capacity of choice. The findings were supported by the existing literature on the specific topic [25, 26] and suggested the following considerations.

First, the MBP was useful to promote the independence and self-determination of a boy with FXS and developmental disabilities. His active role was fostered and the constructive engagement enhanced [27]. Second, the opportunity of choice was corroborated. Henry functionally learned the use of the adaptive responding and varied the inputs according to his preferences [28, 29]. Third, the participant's quality of life was improved as well. Thus, the intervals with indices of happiness increased as sign of an active role [30].

CONCLUSION

Despite the promising data, caution is mandatory because it was a case-report. Generalization was limited accordingly. Furthermore, the equipment included basic technological devices and more sophisticated technological aids to support the participant's complex needs are warranted. A follow-up phase was finally recommended, combined with social validation procedures. In light of the above, future research perspectives should deal with the following topics: (a) extension to new participants with FXS, (b) new extension of the technological solutions, (c) follow-up/generalization phases, and (d) social validation assessments with expert external raters.

REFERENCES

[1] Deng P, Klyachko VA. Channelopathies in fragile X syndrome. *Nat. Rev. Neurosci.* 2021;22(5):275-289.

[2] McLay L, Roche L, France KG, Blampied NM, Lang R, France M, et al. Systematic review of the effectiveness of behaviorally-based interventions for sleep problems in people with rare genetic neurodevelopmental disorders. *Sleep Med. Rev.* 2019; 46:54-63.

[3] Sabus A, Feinstein J, Romani P, Goldson E, Blackmer A. Management of Self-injurious Behaviors in Children with Neurodevelopmental Disorders: A Pharmacotherapy Overview. *Pharmacotherapy* 2019;39(6):645-664.

[4] Jalnapurkar I, Cochran DM, Frazier JA. New Therapeutic Options for Fragile X Syndrome. *Curr. Treat Options Neurol.* 2019;21(3).

[5] Mollajani R, Joghataei MT, Tehrani-Doost M. Review paper: Bumetanide therapeutic effect in children and adolescents with autism spectrum disorder: A review study. *Basic Clin. Neurosci.* 2019;10(5):433-441.

[6] Beresford B, McDaid C, Parker A, Scantlebury A, Spiers G, Fairhurst C, et al. Pharmacological and non-pharmacological interventions for non-respiratory sleep disturbance in children with neurodisabilities: A systematic review. *Health Technol. Assess.* 2018;22(60):1-117.

[7] Hardiman RL, McGill P. How common are challenging behaviours amongst individuals with Fragile X Syndrome? A systematic review. *Res. Dev. Disabil.* 2018; 76:99-109.

[8] Huisman S, Mulder P, Kuijk J, Kerstholt M, van Eeghen A, Leenders A, et al. Self-injurious behavior. *Neurosci. Biobehav. Rev.* 2018; 84:483-491.

[9] Hagerman RJ, Berry-Kravis E, Hazlett HC, Bailey DB, Jr, Moine H, Kooy RF, et al. Fragile X syndrome. *Nat. Rev. Dis. Primers* 2017; 3:17065.

[10] Budimirovic DB, Berry-Kravis E, Erickson CA, Hall SS, Hessl D, Reiss AL, et al. Updated report on tools to measure outcomes of clinical trials in fragile X syndrome. *J. Neurodevelopmental Disord.* 2017;9(1).

[11] Robb N, Northridge J, Politis Y, Zhang B. Parental intention to support the use of computerized cognitive training for children with genetic neurodevelopmental disorders. *Front. Public Health* 2018;6.

[12] Riley K, Bodine C, Hills J, Gane LW, Sandstrum J, Hagerman R. The tickle box assistive technology device piloted on a young woman with fragile X syndrome. *Ment. Health Asp. Dev. Disabil.* 2001;4(4):138-142.

[13] Mirrett PL, Roberts JE, Price J. Early Intervention Practices and Communication Intervention Strategies for Young Males with Fragile X Syndrome. *Lang. Speech Hear Serv. Sch.* 2003;34(4):320-331.

[14] Sequeira AR, Mentzakis E, Archangelidi O, Paolucci F. The economic and health impact of rare diseases: A meta-analysis. *Health Policy Technol.* 2021;10(1):32-44.

[15] Stasolla F, Boccasini A, Perilli V, Caffò AO, Damiani R, Albano V. A selective overview of microswitch-based programs for promoting adaptive behaviors of children with developmental disabilities. *Int. J. Ambient Comput. Intell.* 2014;6(2):56-74.

[16] Stasolla F, Perilli V, Caffò AO, Boccasini A, Stella A, Damiani R, et al. Extending microswitch-cluster programs to promote occupation activities and reduce mouthing by six children with autism spectrum

disorders and intellectual disabilities. *J. Dev. Phys. Disabil.* 2017;29(2):307-324.

[17] Stasolla F, Perilli V, Damiani R, Albano V. Assistive technology to promote occupation and reduce mouthing by three boys with fragile X syndrome. *Dev. Neurorehabilitation* 2017;20(4):185-193.

[18] Stasolla F, Damiani R, Perilli V, Di Leone A, Albano V, Stella A, et al. Technological supports to promote choice opportunities by two children with fragile X syndrome and severe to profound developmental disabilities. *Res. Dev. Disabil.* 2014;35(11):2993-3000.

[19] Sequeira AR, Mentzakis E, Archangelidi O, Paolucci F. The economic and health impact of rare diseases: A meta-analysis. *Health Policy Technol.* 2021;10(1):32-44.

[20] Hall SS, Monlux KD, Rodriguez AB, Jo B, Pollard JS. Telehealth-enabled behavioral treatment for problem behaviors in boys with fragile X syndrome: a randomized controlled trial. *J. Neurodevelopmental Disord.* 2020;12(1).

[21] Crawford MR, Schuster JW. Using microswitches to teach toy use. *J. Dev. Phys. Disabil.* 1993;5(4):349-368.

[22] Stasolla F, Caffò AO, Perilli V, Boccasini A, Stella A, Damiani R, et al. A microswitch-based program for promoting initial ambulation responses: An evaluation with two girls with multiple disabilities. *J. Appl. Behav. Anal.* 2017;50(2):345-356.

[23] Stasolla F, Caffò AO, Perilli V, Boccasini A, Damiani R, Albano V, et al. Comparing self-monitoring and differential reinforcement of an alternative behavior to promote on-task behavior by three children with cerebral palsy: A pilot study. *Life Span Disabil.* 2017;20(1):63-92.

[24] Stasolla F, Perilli V, Boccasini A, Caffò AO, Damiani R, Albano V. Enhancing academic performance of three boys with autism spectrum disorders and intellectual disabilities through a computer-based program. *Life Span Disabil.* 2016;19(2):153-183.

[25] Beresford B, McDaid C, Parker A, Scantlebury A, Spiers G, Fairhurst C, et al. Pharmacological and non-pharmacological

interventions for non-respiratory sleep disturbance in children with neurodisabilities: A systematic review. *Health Technol. Assess.* 2018;22(60):1-117.

[26] Reiss AL, Hall SS. Fragile X Syndrome: Assessment and Treatment Implications. *Child Adolesc. Psychiatr. Clin. North Am.* 2007;16(3):663-675.

[27] Budimirovic DB, Berry-Kravis E, Erickson CA, Hall SS, Hessl D, Reiss AL, et al. Updated report on tools to measure outcomes of clinical trials in fragile X syndrome. *J. Neurodevelopmental Disord.* 2017;9(1).

[28] Dicé F, Auricchio M, Boursier V, De Luca Picione R, Santamaria F, Salerno M, et al. Psychological Scaffolding for taking charge of Intersex/DSD conditions. The Joint Listening Settings. *Psicol. Salute* 2018;2018(1):129-145.

[29] Freda MF, Savarese L, Bova M, Galante A, De Falco R, De Luca Picione R, et al. Stress and Psychological Factors in the Variable Clinical Phenotype of Hereditary Angioedema in Children: A Pilot Study. Pediatr. *Allergy Immunol. Pulmonol.* 2016;29(1):6-12.

[30] Stasolla F, Caffò AO, Perilli V, Albano V. Experimental Examination and Social Validation of a Microswitch Intervention to Improve Choice-Making and Activity Engagement for Six Girls with Rett Syndrome. *Dev. Neurorehabilitation* 2019;22(8):527-541.

ABOUT THE EDITOR

Fabrizio Stasolla is an Associate Professor of Developmental Psychology at "Giustino Fortunato" University of Benevento (Italy). His interests deal with assistive technology-based programs and rehabilitative interventions to promote an active role, independence, and self-determination in individuals with neurological disorders and severe to profound and multiple disabilities. Additionally, he is interested in aided-alternative and augmentative communication strategies to support communication skills in non-verbal individuals. Recently, he fits virtual reality setups, new and wearable technologies, and telerehabilitation for both assessment and recovery purposes in persons with neurodevelopmental disorders and neurodegenerative diseases. Furthermore, patients with acquired brain injuries either in a vegetative state, in a minimally conscious state or emerging/emerged from it are usually targeted along his research interests. Children with attention deficit hyperactivity disorders, autism spectrum disorders, cerebral palsy, rare genetic diseases, Alzheimer's or Parkinson's diseases, amyotrophic lateral sclerosis or lateral sclerosis are finally included. On that specific topic, he authored several international papers published in peer-reviewed Journals. He also edited *Understanding Children with Cerebral Palsy* (NOVA Publisher, 2020) and actually he is in the process of editing one forthcoming NOVA volume entitled *A Clinical Guide to Cerebral Palsy*. Moreover, he recently edited a new IGI Global volume entitled *Assistive Technologies for Assessment and Recovery of Neurological Impairments*. Finally, he is an Associate Editor for Frontiers in Psychology (Neuropsychology Section).

INDEX

A

academic performance, 143, 157
adaptive response, 112, 114, 117, 120, 122, 123, 124, 137, 138, 139, 140, 142, 151, 152, 153
adolescents, 24, 38, 47, 69, 74, 78, 82, 91, 98, 114, 135, 155
adults, 2, 24, 25, 76, 80, 81, 89, 90, 97, 126, 130, 131
adverse effects, xi, 62, 65, 75, 77
aggression, ix, xi, 22, 47, 54, 58, 67, 68, 69, 74, 78, 94, 99, 100, 113, 135, 137, 149, 150
aggressive and self-injurious behaviors, 63
aggressive behavior, 53, 68, 78, 99
amygdala, 19, 37, 96, 102
antipsychotic, 68, 69, 78, 85
anxiety, x, 9, 16, 17, 22, 23, 44, 45, 47, 48, 50, 51, 54, 56, 57, 59, 63, 64, 66, 67, 68, 69, 73, 74, 78, 79, 84, 85, 93, 94, 98, 100, 102, 106, 111, 113, 137, 150

anxiety disorders, 44, 47, 51, 56, 57, 59, 66, 84, 85, 106
assessment, 45, 89, 106, 108, 114, 125, 129, 142, 146, 159
assistive technology, x, xii, 112, 113, 122, 123, 125, 126, 127, 129, 131, 134, 135, 143, 145, 146, 148, 149, 156, 157, 159
assistive technology-based interventions, x, 113, 135, 149
ataxia, 2, 4, 6, 8, 9, 29, 143
attention deficit and hyperactivity disorder (ADHD), 22, 44, 45, 47, 49, 52, 57, 63, 64, 65, 67, 78, 83, 102
autism, ix, x, 4, 9, 22, 30, 34, 38, 43, 44, 45, 46, 47, 48, 49, 53, 54, 56, 58, 59, 64, 67, 81, 82, 84, 85, 86, 87, 88, 99, 102, 104, 105, 106, 107, 108, 113, 127, 128, 129, 130, 142, 143, 155, 156, 157, 159
avoidance, 48, 74, 79, 93, 98, 105, 108, 113
awareness, xii, 45, 148, 153

B

behavioral alterations, 49, 64
behavioral change, 74, 100
behavioral manifestations, 45
behavioral problems, 22, 65, 148
behaviors, xi, 19, 22, 27, 46, 53, 54, 62, 63, 67, 68, 69, 78, 79, 93, 94, 98, 99, 100, 101, 102, 107, 112, 113, 114, 115, 118, 122, 123, 124, 127, 129, 135, 140, 143, 149, 156
beneficial effect, 26, 73, 122, 125
brain, xi, 2, 3, 4, 10, 12, 15, 17, 19, 23, 27, 29, 31, 34, 69, 70, 71, 77, 84, 90, 94, 95, 96, 98, 104, 113, 159
brain size, 96
brain structure, xi, 77, 94, 95, 96, 101
brainstem, 143
breast cancer, 20
burden reduction, 149

C

cancer, 17, 20, 21, 38, 39, 40, 89
cancer progression, 20, 21, 38, 39
cancer stem cells, 39
cancer therapy, 40
caregivers, x, xii, 54, 74, 95, 106, 115, 116, 123, 125, 137, 149
catatonia, x, 44, 46, 52, 55
cell body, 10, 12
cell cycle, 4, 20, 33
cell line, 11, 20, 39
cell signaling, 71
cerebellum, 10, 15, 23, 24, 143
cerebral palsy, 135, 146, 157, 159
CGG repeats, 2, 5, 6, 8, 45
challenges, 45, 46, 113, 135, 145
challenging behavior, xi, 58, 62, 94, 95, 98, 99, 101, 103, 107, 112, 114, 117, 119, 120, 122, 123, 124, 125, 130, 135

childhood, 9, 64, 66, 69, 126
children, 7, 24, 25, 38, 45, 47, 48, 49, 50, 51, 52, 57, 58, 62, 64, 65, 67, 69, 70, 73, 74, 76, 77, 78, 81, 82, 83, 84, 86, 90, 91, 97, 100, 101, 104, 105, 108, 112, 114, 115, 116, 117, 122, 123, 125, 126, 127, 128, 129, 143, 145, 146, 155, 156, 157, 158
choice capacities, 149
circadian rhythm, 58, 70, 74
clinical presentation, xi, 8, 44, 49, 54, 87
clinical trials, 24, 35, 75, 128, 156, 158
cognition, 46, 50, 77, 78, 80, 87, 96
cognitive activity, 100
cognitive deficits, x, 8, 44, 46, 73, 89
cognitive dysfunction, 142
cognitive flexibility, 25
cognitive function, xi, 62, 63, 67
cognitive level, 103
cognitive performance, 16, 17
cognitive skills, 45
cognitive-behavioral programs, 149
communication, 48, 93, 97, 102, 103, 104, 116, 127, 131, 134, 135, 136, 145, 149, 159
communication interactions, 135
comorbidities, xi, 44, 45, 47, 48, 54, 55, 62, 64
constructive engagement, vii, xii, 111, 113, 117, 125, 128, 129, 134, 135, 140, 141, 149, 150, 154
containers, xii, 114, 151, 152, 153
control group, 46, 47, 49, 73
controlled trials, 25, 67, 80
cytoplasm, 3, 14, 21
cytosine, 45, 63, 102
cytoskeleton, 3, 11, 32

D

defects, 18, 23, 41, 71, 74, 90

deficiency, 43, 45, 70
deficit, x, 3, 5, 9, 22, 44, 45, 49, 54, 57, 59, 74, 82, 83, 84, 159
dendrites, x, 2, 3, 4, 5, 12, 27
dendritic spines, 3, 12, 15, 17, 36, 70, 87
dependent variable, 123
depression, 13, 15, 23, 33, 50, 51, 67, 73, 79, 102
depressive disorder, 9, 50, 51
depressive symptoms, 78, 85
development on pathological mechanisms, 4
developmental and intellectual disabilities, 116, 148
developmental disabilities, vii, viii, ix, 94, 100, 103, 104, 105, 107, 109, 111, 112, 113, 114, 115, 126, 127, 128, 129, 130, 133, 134, 135, 136, 142, 143, 144, 145, 147, 148, 150, 154, 156, 157
developmental disorder, 127
disability, x, 1, 2, 3, 4, 22, 44, 45, 47, 54, 68, 97, 98, 102, 103, 129
disease progression, 20
disorder, x, 4, 43, 44, 45, 47, 49, 50, 51, 54, 56, 57, 59, 63, 78, 82, 83, 84, 93, 94, 97, 107, 112, 155
DNA, x, 14, 27, 33, 95, 116, 136, 150
DNA damage, 14, 33
dopamine, 13, 64, 65, 78
dopaminergic, 67, 68, 69
Drosophila, 8, 9, 18, 23, 33, 38, 41, 73, 75, 77, 88, 89, 90
drug targets, 36, 63
drug therapy, 100
drug treatment, 64, 68
drugs, 7, 26, 65, 66, 83, 86, 100

E

economic consequences, 106
environmental factors, 54, 100, 101

epilepsy, ix, xi, 17, 44, 54, 135
equipment, 113, 135, 149, 155
evidence, xi, 10, 14, 20, 30, 46, 51, 54, 62, 64, 71, 97, 99, 103, 122, 126
excitatory synapses, 17, 22
executive function, x, 9, 44, 46, 96, 97
experimental condition, 118, 119, 137, 140, 151
experimental design, 128, 138, 141, 148, 152
external environment, 113
external validity, 125
extracellular matrix, 19

F

families, x, 22, 51, 54, 81, 149
FMR1, ix, x, 2, 3, 4, 5, 6, 7, 8, 9, 10, 11, 12, 13, 15, 16, 17, 18, 19, 22, 23, 24, 27, 28, 29, 30, 31, 35, 37, 40, 41, 45, 50, 51, 53, 56, 57, 62, 63, 71, 74, 76, 77, 93, 94, 95, 96, 97, 98, 102, 108, 113, 135, 148
FMR1 gene, ix, x, 2, 3, 4, 5, 6, 7, 8, 9, 10, 11, 22, 27, 28, 29, 45, 56, 62, 93, 94, 97, 98, 102, 108, 135, 148
FMRP, x, 1, 2, 3, 4, 5, 6, 8, 9, 10, 11, 12, 13, 14, 15, 16, 17, 18, 19, 20, 21, 22, 23, 27, 30, 31, 32, 33, 34, 39, 40, 45, 63, 70, 71, 80, 81, 87, 88, 95, 96, 98, 101, 102, 104
formation, 16, 19, 20, 32, 38, 39
fragile x syndrome, 38, 81, 84, 91, 94
fragile X syndrome, vii, viii, ix, x, xi, xii, 1, 2, 3, 4, 6, 7, 9, 22, 25, 26, 27, 28, 29, 30, 31, 32, 33, 34, 35, 36, 37, 38, 39, 40, 41, 43, 44, 45, 55, 56, 57, 58, 59, 61, 62, 63, 71, 72, 78, 81, 82, 83, 84, 85, 86, 87, 88, 89, 90, 91, 93, 94, 101, 102, 103, 104, 105, 106, 107, 108, 111, 112, 114, 115, 126, 127, 128, 129, 130, 133, 134,

135, 143, 145, 147, 148, 155, 156, 157, 158
functional occupation, viii, 147, 148, 149

G

gene expression, 4, 45
genes, 4, 18, 21, 26, 39, 45, 58, 90
genetic disease, ix, 111, 135, 159
genetic disorders, 56
glutamate, 11, 13, 14, 15, 16, 18, 24, 25, 27, 32, 35, 63, 71, 72, 75, 100
glutamate receptor antagonists, 27
growth, 13, 16, 17, 23, 71
growth factor, 13, 71
guanine, 21, 45, 63, 102

H

happiness, 115, 118, 130, 141, 148, 150, 151, 153, 154
headache, 24, 78, 79
health, 63, 156, 157
hepatocellular carcinoma, 20, 39
hippocampus, 15, 19, 23, 34, 35, 37, 76, 87
human, 10, 15, 19, 20, 29, 36, 41
hyperactive and/or autistic behavior, 3
hyperactivity, ix, x, 15, 19, 22, 24, 25, 44, 45, 47, 49, 53, 54, 57, 59, 63, 64, 66, 75, 78, 79, 82, 83, 84, 93, 107, 113, 135, 149, 159

I

impairments, 48, 63, 67, 69, 73, 93, 97, 134, 135, 136
improvements, 24, 74, 75, 77, 79, 80, 84
impulsivity, 47, 49, 93, 94, 99, 111, 149
independence, x, 80, 95, 123, 134, 149, 154, 159

indices of happiness, 115, 118, 130, 141, 148, 150, 151, 153, 154
individuals, x, xi, xii, 3, 13, 22, 25, 39, 44, 47, 51, 52, 53, 58, 59, 62, 63, 64, 66, 67, 68, 69, 70, 73, 74, 75, 76, 77, 80, 95, 96, 97, 99, 100, 101, 102, 103, 105, 106, 107, 108, 109, 113, 126, 129, 130, 135, 149, 156, 159
inhibition, 15, 24, 25, 35, 37, 38, 48, 67, 74, 78, 79, 88
inhibitor, 24, 25, 76, 78, 80
injury, iv, xi, 53, 54, 78, 94, 100, 135
intellectual development, xi, 50, 94, 95, 97, 101, 104
intellectual disability, x, 1, 2, 3, 4, 44, 45, 46, 47, 54, 68, 97, 98, 102, 103, 107, 108, 129
intelligence quotient, 46, 97
intervention, ix, xi, xii, 25, 62, 63, 76, 84, 86, 90, 95, 99, 103, 112, 114, 115, 116, 117, 118, 119, 120, 121, 122, 124, 127, 134, 137, 138, 139, 140, 141, 151, 152, 154
intervention strategies, 62, 127
intracellular calcium, 75
irritability, 24, 25, 65, 68, 69, 74, 78
isolation, 32, 93, 123, 141, 147, 150
issues, xi, 8, 63, 94, 95, 108

L

language development, xi, 62, 67, 73, 78, 102
learning, x, 3, 5, 14, 22, 34, 35, 44, 46, 50, 53, 54, 63, 70, 73, 80, 86, 87, 93, 94, 97, 101, 102, 113, 123, 124, 135, 139
learning and memory, 3, 5, 70, 87
learning difficulties, 50, 93, 94, 97, 113, 135
learning disabilities, xi, 44, 53, 54, 86, 97
learning process, 124, 139

light, 115, 118, 120, 142, 149, 155

M

management, 28, 29, 55, 63, 68, 69, 80, 82, 123
manipulation, xi, 35, 104, 113, 115, 117, 129, 136, 137, 139
matrix metalloproteinase, 15, 36, 38, 71, 90
medical, 36, 52, 55, 63, 73, 95, 108, 123
medication, ix, 65, 68, 73, 75, 79, 80
melatonin, 52, 58, 70, 78, 86, 87
memory, ix, 3, 5, 9, 23, 35, 50, 68, 70, 74, 87, 97
mental retardation, ix, 1, 26, 27, 28, 29, 30, 31, 32, 33, 34, 38, 41, 43, 45, 50, 63, 86, 88, 95
metabolism, 11, 16, 20, 21, 28, 32, 37, 40, 80
mice, 12, 13, 15, 16, 17, 18, 19, 23, 35, 37, 41, 71, 74, 76, 87
microswitches, 113, 117, 124, 128, 135, 137, 142, 144, 157
molecules, 4, 25, 38, 71, 72, 100
mood change, 67, 78
mood disorder, ix, xi, 52, 62, 67
mood swings, x, 44, 45
mRNA, 2, 3, 4, 5, 6, 8, 10, 11, 12, 13, 14, 15, 16, 19, 20, 21, 23, 27, 30, 31, 32, 33, 35, 38, 40, 104
mutation, ix, x, xi, 5, 11, 29, 31, 44, 45, 46, 49, 54, 56, 59, 63, 93, 95, 98, 104, 116, 148, 150
mutations, 45, 46, 90, 148

N

neurobiology, 22, 34
neuroblastoma, 12
neurodegeneration, 8, 70
neurodegenerative diseases, 159

neurodevelopmental disorders, 40, 48, 52, 57, 70, 145, 155, 156, 159
neurons, 4, 11, 12, 14, 19, 22, 30, 32, 33, 71, 76
neuropsychiatric conditions, 44, 45
nucleus, 3, 4, 14, 21, 78, 96, 102

P

parents, xii, 49, 52, 95, 99, 101, 114, 115, 116, 123, 125, 134, 137, 138, 141, 146, 150, 151
participants, 53, 76, 112, 114, 115, 116, 117, 118, 119, 122, 123, 124, 125, 136, 138, 142, 149, 155
pathway, 14, 16, 20, 25, 26, 37, 65, 71, 78, 79
permutated phenotypes, 2
pharmacological treatment, ix, 55, 62, 63, 64, 65, 100, 102
pharmacotherapy, vii, xi, 36, 61, 62, 64, 83, 85, 155
phenotype, xi, 2, 5, 6, 11, 15, 23, 41, 45, 47, 54, 58, 59, 63, 69, 74, 76, 80, 86, 94, 95, 98, 99, 107, 135, 142, 143
placebo, 25, 38, 67, 73, 76, 81, 83, 84, 85, 91
population, 5, 7, 28, 47, 48, 51, 54, 64, 65, 113, 149
positive interactions, 95
positive mood, 115, 150, 154
positive participation, xii, 112, 113, 114, 119, 121, 122, 124, 135, 140, 141, 148, 149, 150
post-transcriptional regulation, 3, 5
post-traumatic stress disorder, 51
premutation carriers, 5, 29, 30, 53, 57, 59
problem behavior, 106, 107, 108, 157
protein synthesis, 4, 11, 13, 15, 23, 35, 76, 90

proteins, x, 2, 3, 4, 8, 11, 12, 15, 16, 18, 19, 25, 31, 40, 63, 80
psychiatric disorder, 70, 102, 143
psychological problems, 101
psychologist, 116, 136, 150

Q

quality of life, x, 22, 81, 95, 112, 114, 122, 128, 129, 134, 135, 141, 148, 149, 150, 154

R

rare genetic disease, ix, 111, 159
receptor, 12, 13, 14, 15, 16, 18, 20, 22, 23, 25, 27, 32, 35, 63, 65, 71, 72, 76, 78, 79, 85, 87, 88
repetitive behavior, 23, 24, 52, 53, 99, 100, 105
response, 4, 13, 14, 23, 24, 33, 47, 48, 69, 75, 78, 112, 114, 117, 123, 124, 136, 138, 139, 141, 151, 152, 153
restricted and repetitive behavior, 52
risk, 6, 7, 20, 28, 39, 48, 51, 53, 65, 66, 67, 76, 99
risk factors, 51, 99
RNA, 3, 4, 5, 10, 11, 12, 14, 17, 19, 20, 21, 28, 29, 30, 31, 32, 34, 40

S

seizures and abnormalities in electroencephalogram, 51
self-injury behavior, xi, 53, 54, 135
signaling pathway, 5, 13, 20, 33, 64, 88
sleep disorders, 3, 52, 58, 63, 70
sleep disturbance, 9, 66, 78, 86, 155, 158
small intestine, 10
social anxiety, 48, 56, 67

social communication, xi, 48, 94, 95, 97, 101
social communication difficulties, 48
social environment, 101
social image, 95, 123, 135
social impairment, 78
social interaction, ix, xii, 49, 53, 98, 108, 134, 136, 138, 139, 140, 141
social interactions, ix, xii, 49, 98, 134, 136, 138
social withdrawal, xi, 25, 44, 47, 49, 54
special education, ix, 116, 136
speech, ix, 24, 25, 116, 137, 150
spine, 8, 15, 16, 17, 32, 36, 73, 91
stimulation, xii, 17, 99, 101, 113, 114, 118, 119, 123, 124, 128, 134, 135, 136, 137, 139, 141, 144, 149, 151, 153
stress, 13, 14, 50, 52, 70, 99
symptoms, x, 9, 22, 23, 46, 47, 49, 50, 53, 55, 56, 63, 64, 65, 66, 67, 68, 69, 70, 74, 78, 79, 80, 85, 100, 102, 106, 148
synaptic plasticity, 3, 5, 10, 15, 17, 27, 30, 33, 35, 40, 70, 71, 79, 88
synthesis, x, 2, 5, 12, 13, 15, 18, 27, 71, 76, 86

T

target, x, xi, 2, 5, 15, 18, 20, 23, 27, 36, 40, 54, 62, 71, 72, 80, 87
targeted treatments, xi, 40, 62, 63, 64, 71, 72, 77, 80, 81, 82, 87, 129
theoretical approach, 100
therapy, ix, 34, 40, 65, 75, 84
translation, x, 2, 4, 8, 11, 12, 13, 15, 17, 19, 21, 23, 28, 31, 32, 33, 34, 35, 102
transport, 4, 12, 14, 21, 33
treatment, xi, 2, 4, 8, 15, 16, 19, 22, 24, 25, 26, 34, 37, 41, 44, 55, 62, 63, 64, 65, 66, 67, 68, 69, 70, 71, 73, 74, 75, 76, 77, 78,

80, 81, 82, 83, 84, 85, 87, 89, 90, 91, 102, 103, 104, 106, 107, 126, 157, 158
tremor, 2, 4, 6, 8, 9, 29, 78, 143
trial, 24, 25, 38, 67, 69, 73, 74, 75, 76, 77, 81, 83, 85, 90, 91, 157

weight gain, 67, 69
weight loss, 67, 73, 79, 84, 85
white matter, 8, 9, 11, 96
withdrawal, 66, 95, 141, 149, 150
work activities, 126, 128, 130
working memory, ix, x, 25, 44, 46, 50

V

validation, 31, 114, 125, 142, 144, 146, 155
videos, 117, 118, 119, 151, 152, 153
VOCA, viii, xii, 133, 134, 136, 137, 138, 139, 140, 141, 144

X

X chromosome, ix, 7, 26, 93, 94, 98, 102, 135, 148

Y

young adults, 24, 25, 83, 129

W

weight control, 74